Tragedy to Triumph

The Story of Tom's Heart

Janet W. Mauk and Pete Radigan
as told to Jim McGrath

Red Penguin
BOOKS

This book encompassed a labor of love, rich powerful memories, and strong emotions that surrounded the tragedy and loss interwoven with the power of hope. We cannot thank our family and friends enough, far too many to mention, for your unending support throughout our personal, intimate, individual, and collective journeys together. Your listening ears and words of encouragement contributed to our healing and enabled us to provide hope for others who have, who are, or who will be traveling this road. In our minds, you made this story possible and have our profound gratitude.

And to my beloved son, Thomas Corbin, whose thoughtful plan and loving decision made this possible. There is a gift in every tragedy which he wanted to share. I loved all that you were for 16 years, 345 days and 20 hours on earth—which went far too fast. I miss our talks and miss being your mom!

Contents

Prologue

A Big Heart

I met Pete Radigan in the mid-1990s when he became a patient in my Internal Medicine practice. Pete was a bright, hard-working young man ready to take on all the opportunities and challenges life had in store for him. Pete was also a kind, caring, giving, and conscientious person, always willing to take an extra step for the benefit of others. Within hours of meeting Pete, I knew that he had such a big heart.

In the late 1990s, we learned that Pete's heart was too large, the result of an uncommon disease. Pete was diagnosed with severe cardiomyopathy (a heart muscle disease) that rapidly developed into Stage 4 heart failure. This was end-stage heart failure. Pete was going to die unless he received a heart transplant.

Throughout the years, I cared for Pete before his transplant; and despite the continuous bad news about the progression of his disease, he sustained a positive attitude. He remained gracious, optimistic, and determined to fight his medical challenges. It was an honor and a pleasure to care for such a strong, kind, and admirable patient. Pete sat in the hospital for months waiting and hoping for a transplant. Despite being bedridden, his kindness and optimism never flagged.

Eventually, we received the news that a suitable heart had been found, and Pete went into surgery. The procedure, mercifully, went as well as could be hoped.

After his successful transplantation, Pete remained the giving, kind man he is, eager to help others and to make a positive impact on the world. He gave back to his community by working with Transplant Speakers International, whose mission is to raise awareness and to educate the public about organ and tissue donation. He continued to live his life to the fullest, making the most of every day with a deep appreciation of the gift he received.

Pete felt a deep need to connect to the family of his donor after his transplant. He was so grateful for the gift he had received, but this gratitude was tempered with the understanding that his gift of life was due to the loss of another. He wanted to thank his donor's family for this sacrifice and gift. And so, he did.

A year after his procedure, with the consent of both parties, Pete met his donor's mother, Janet Mauk. They formed a beautiful, respectful relationship, a true friendship that has lasted now for over 20 years. This extraordinary journey, in the pages ahead, is their story, told from both of their perspectives. It is a demonstration of the power of love, hope, generosity, kindness, and friendship, along with the astonishing power that transplant medicine provides to save lives.

- Lynne Becker Kossow, MD

PART I

Janet's Story

1

Janet's Younger Son

Tom Mauk packed his bags. It was time to go. As the second son of divorced parents, he had made the best of living with his mom, Janet, but even she knew he was serious this time. As he approached his 13th birthday, the youngster tired of the weekend visits with his father, sought his camaraderie, and was ready to make the move a permanent one.

For months he had broached the topic with his mother, but she attempted to change the conversation. As she recalled later in her journal, "I did not want to face that possibility." At other times, we freely discussed the benefits and drawbacks. Tom remained persistent in returning to the subject. Today she was seeing it with her own eyes. Tom was a teenager, now 13, and felt ready to make this decision without interference.

"I'll never forget getting up from a nap and seeing Tom's bags packed," wrote Janet. "At first, I thought he had not yet unpacked from his visit with his father."

Then Tom said, "I want to go and live with my father."

She replied, "Does your father know about it?"

He said, "Yes, I told him."

She knew now that he would never give up on the subject. He had made up his mind. However, Janet was not ready to relinquish her younger son. She picked up the phone to call his father, only to find out he was equally surprised. "I thought Tom was teasing," his father quipped. "I didn't think he was serious."

Janet thought she was prepared to face reality. She knew at that age it was not unusual for boys with divorced parents to reside with their father. In her mind, many children needed to experience living with their fathers, much to the chagrin of some mothers. In many cases, dads earn more money, and the child hopes he will buy them nice things. Some feel safer with their fathers. Some seek a more permissive lifestyle with few or no boundaries. Sometimes they seek the continuous fun they experienced during visitations. But as Janet talked with Tom's father on the phone, her protective mothering stance came to the forefront and she adamantly retorted, "If you want him, you are going to have to fight for him!"

Reflecting later, Janet knew that several areas bothered her as she pondered the possibility of Tom moving. He had qualified for special education services in third grade due to his diagnosis of Attention-Deficit Disorder (ADD) and consistently struggled with formal education. The results of IQ tests revealed an above-average intelligence, but somehow, attempting to conform to the mold of formal education was like putting a square peg in a round hole. He enjoyed attending school but learned in his own unique, God-given way. Throughout his elementary years, Janet learned that a structured environment, taking Ritalin, and being in a self-contained classroom proved to be Tom's formula for consistent academic progress. An individualized educational program (IEP) had already been initiated. An IEP is a map outlining a program of special education instruction which includes support and services children need in order to continue their progress and thrive in school. This is developed by the Special Education team with support from the parents. Tom's ADD became a constant challenge to manage at home and school.

Jan had invested a great deal of time and energy in his pursuits, taking advantage of the support available, and feared the results of these efforts would be squelched in a rural school through limited resources and assistance. She had previously educated herself in the field of special education and volunteered as a special education advocate in the city schools.

A secondary concern involved Tom being alone at night without supervision due to his father's work schedule of 11:00 p.m. to 7:00 a.m. She knew even though teenagers complain to their parents about certain boundaries, they indeed feel secure knowing they exist. She discussed these concerns openly with both Tom and his father, but his father had a roommate at that time, so Tom would not be alone. On his end, Tom's father was willing to try it and felt, if necessary, he could work during the day.

Janet had raised Tom to recognize the value of attending church on a regular basis. She understood its importance in her life and attempted to teach it in the lives of her boys, as well. Tom enjoyed attending church and worshipping God and usually attended without prodding. She hoped he would continue to follow this practice after his move.

She did not regret her verbal challenge to Tom's father and sought legal advice but did not receive the legal feedback she expected. Despite genuine concerns, the attorney told her that unless she was able to prove that Tom's father could not hold a job, the judge would probably honor Tom's request, since at 13 years of age he could legally choose. He stated, "You could probably spend a few thousand dollars, but there is no guarantee we would win."

Jan reminded herself that her children were on loan from God as she faced the reality of losing her son. She would have to trust God with her precious child and her concerns.

On the way to church one Sunday, Tom shared his heart with his mother. "Mom, I'm going to my father's because I need to be with him, not because you are a bad mother." As Janet later recalled in her journal, Tom displayed perception beyond his years and always articulated it well. It seemed he could read her soul. Janet did not want to deny him being with his father. He could certainly fill needs in Tom's life that she could not.

Janet struggled with her son's anticipated move until one day when she realized that God works all things out and that He is bigger than the situation. She consoled herself knowing Tom would only be living 34 miles away and that she could visit him anytime.

At the time, it appeared Tom was making the biggest decision of his young life. Little did she know what the future would hold.

In November of 1993, Janet awarded custody of Tom to his father. Tom had finished his first ten weeks of the seventh grade with her in Niagara Falls, New York. As he prepared to move, she sent and discussed Tom's records with the special education leaders at his new school, specifically focusing on Tom's learning style. He then transitioned from a self-contained classroom in Niagara Falls where he continued to make consistent progress to a consulting model at the rural school. The difference between the two is that a self-contained classroom consists of a special education teacher and several students with similar academic, social, and emotional needs who each have an IEP, while a consulting model consists of students with similar academic, social, or emotional needs who attend classes with the general population. The students return to the classroom for extra help from the consultant teacher educated in special education. Janet began to feel uncomfortable and reluctant regarding this approach and questioned its validity for Tom.

Tom wanted to fit in with his peers and not be labeled "different," yet Janet lacked the confidence that he could survive educationally. He refused to take his prescribed Ritalin, and she anticipated more struggles. Questioning Tom's potential success, she offered no input for a while, realizing his father needed to experience some of Tom's struggles.

Tom continued to develop behavior problems due to his academic difficulties, which was no surprise to Jan. Per recommendation by the special education team, Tom transferred to a self-contained classroom at another school for eighth grade. This held promise and he flourished as he survived best in this type of learning environment. Even Janet had to admit it was probably his best year of school to date. She noticed that he seemed more relaxed, more confident of himself, and had demonstrated consistent progress. She was proud of his achievements.

Jan attempted to stay optimistic but feared future troubles would snowball. However, it did not happen immediately. Jan frequently offered and begged Tom to return to the city schools and move back, confident of more educational options, but he continually refused.

The burning question became—how well would Tom handle high school? The Mauk family was about to find out.

High School

The following year, the entire Special Education department returned to his rural school district. The school had developed its own self-contained classroom for high school. At first, Janet felt encouraged by this move and hoped he would again thrive in his preferred learning environment.

It did not take long to realize that the students chosen for this special education class were too diverse in background and academic levels to learn optimally. With more severe needs among many students, they presented a challenge for even the most seasoned teacher.

Janet's continued motherly concern involved Tom's educational survival. She hoped he would have another year like the previous one. Yet, problems loomed from the beginning of Tom's ninth-grade year. In one instance, due to many unforeseen circumstances, Tom experienced three different teachers within a 15-week span. Tom did not fit into any program. Finally, it was suggested he be placed in a consulting model with 19 other students and a consulting teacher. He would be mainstreamed into all the major academic areas, attending classes with the general population. However, in the state of New York, the goal was to provide advanced subject material to prepare students to pass the New York State Regents. In the city schools, students could choose a Regents or a non-Regents path. At the rural school, only one choice was offered.

Janet shared his learning concerns with her sisters who were teachers. They informed her that transitioning from the eighth grade to the ninth grade can be challenging because any academic deficits will show up. Tom's deficiencies came into sharp focus. He lacked confidence in working independently, showed a low level of initiative, and required a great deal of help in completing assignments. He also neglected most of his homework. He only passed two courses that year: English and Gym. Janet felt sad about it, especially knowing he still longed to be like the other students, attend the same classes like the others, and did not want to be different or labeled.

Coupled with his academic shortcomings, Tom refused to take his prescribed Ritalin consistently. She strongly encouraged Tom to take his Ritalin, sharing the difference it made in his everyday life. He was not convinced. He wanted to avoid the embarrassment of going to the nurse before lunch to get his medicine, risking the fact that other students may wonder why he was there. Janet suggested to Tom's father that he request from Tom's primary care physician a prescription for a long-acting Ritalin so that he could avoid daily visits to the nurse. Jan even attempted to advocate in reaching Tom's medical doctor. Tom did not want to accept the fact he had specific and documented learning challenges.

But Janet continued to pray and hope for the best. In the spring of Tom's ninth-grade year, her prayers were answered as she formulated an idea and hoped for Tom's approval.

Excerpts from Janet's Journal:

Summer School 1996

As Tom continued to struggle with his studies, a passage from Janet's journal reflects her concern and determination to have him succeed.

"As Tom's performance in school plummeted, I strongly convinced him to return to Niagara Falls to take Social Studies and Math in summer school. In May of that year, I also signed him up to take tutoring classes at the Sylvan Learning Center. I drove Tom long distances for several months so he could attend tutoring sessions twice a week.

During the first week of summer school, I realized Tom could really learn the concise material and do the work. He started out with a bang, getting good grades, but maintaining them did not seem important to him. He attended school every day and enjoyed socializing and learning. In the end, he did pass both courses. I remember walking five times around "Goat Island," an island surrounding the Niagara River, and begging God to help him pass the state math exam. All students in New York state needed to pass this test in order to graduate from high school. I felt elated and thankful when I returned to school to pick him up and found out that he passed! He felt elated that he passed Social Studies and Math, plus the state exam, and could now start 10th grade. I loved having him live with me for those six weeks. It seemed like he never moved away."

Tom Learns to Drive

Tom's independence began to develop in various forms. As Janet recalled in her journal:

"He would drive my car up and down the driveway, getting ready to earn his permit in a few weeks. He would beg me at times to let him drive in the street, but I adamantly put a stop to it. Sometimes, I would take him on a remote back road and let him drive. He felt excited about taking the test and hopefully having wheels. Since Tom was a year older than most students, he was able to drive in 10th grade since most students do not drive until 11th grade.

He had saved some money and convinced me I needed to take it out of the bank so he could buy a very inexpensive car, work on it, and eventually drive it. After discussing it with his father, I felt convinced it would be a great opportunity for learning since Tom and his father possess natural abilities in mechanics and could work on it together. I allowed him to take the money out of the bank to buy the car. He felt ecstatic and talked nonstop about it.

On his 16th birthday, I took him to the Department of Motor Vehicles in Lockport where he passed the written test to obtain his driving permit. He could not contain his excitement as his father met us there and they left together."

Starting 10th Grade

Armed with a sense of growing independence, Tom appeared excited about returning to school, knowing he could now be in 10th grade. Once again, the special education committee recommended a consulting teacher with 19 other students; in fact, he had the same teacher as the year before.

However, the course material was being taught on a higher level to prepare students to pass the New York State Regents exam at the end of the year. Even though Tom had a caring consultant teacher, I feared the expectations and material would overwhelm him. I knew Tom needed more time and attention than the teacher could give him.

Outside of school, things appeared bleak. Tom signed up for his road test to get his driver's license three weeks after getting his learner's permit. In a minor setback, he failed it the first time. Persistence prevailed but not immediately. Tom signed up again for another test, scheduled two weeks later. Again, he failed. I had not been informed of his choices or I would have discouraged him until he received more experience on the road.

Tom remained determined but not wise. A few weeks later, I received a phone call from his teacher asking if I knew that Tom drove to school without a license. I replied, "No, I didn't know." Even though I had spoken to Tom about driving without a license, he persisted.

When Tom visited on the weekends, he brought his homework which I helped him complete. Yet, his grades continued to plummet. I wanted to save him from the inevitable outcome of failing school but tried not to give up. His educational options were dwindling. It seemed evident the constant transitions he experienced in his academic programs would further add insult to injury.

Quitting School

Frustrated by school, Tom started searching for a way out. However, his mother refused to give up. Just before the Thanksgiving break, she and Tom's father agreed to meet with the Special Education Committee, review Tom's IEP, and further discuss educational options. Even though there are positive benefits in exploring other educational options, some students, and especially their parents, resist following an IEP due to the perceived stigma attached to being a special education student.

Although Jan strongly encouraged Tom to consider returning to Niagara Falls many times for more educational options, he continued to adamantly refuse. Janet retained a degree of optimism, yet she still felt powerless to serve as an advocate. There was one other bit of information she did not know. Her son, already a headstrong individual, had already made up his mind about his educational future and had not shared it with his mom.

He attended the meeting, but it was here that he planned to break the news.

"I plan to quit school!" declared Tom to the group, which included his parents, the Special Education Committee, the counselor, two classroom teachers, and the principal.

Janet's heart sank. If only she could convince Tom of a viable alternative. Perhaps taking afternoon classes and earning a GED? Job-related training? Anything!

The principal, properly versed in these matters, discussed other academic options with Tom, but he refused them all.

"So, what do you plan on doing?" asked the school counselor.

"I plan to pursue employment and work for a living."

The conversation transferred back to his parents.

"How do you as parents feel about this?" asked the principal.

Janet told the committee she disagreed with Tom quitting school, but she knew the Regents track course content was too difficult and Tom needed more realistic options. Jan knew the decision was out of her hands because in New York state children can choose to quit school when they turn 16. She felt powerless. Although Tom's father agreed that Tom should stay in school, he stated, "But these days, children have more rights than parents." It appeared the principal's attempt to advocate for Tom's need was to no avail as the principal expressed frustration.

Janet knew the struggles that awaited Tom. She realized he had lost a lot academically by moving and changing schools. She worried that perhaps too much water had gone over the dam! Her son could not keep up with the Regents program. It was a human impossibility!

Tom stood up in a very polite manner and asked the principal what he would have to do to quit school. In a strange way, Janet felt proud of him for demonstrating confidence yet developed a sickening feeling inside. She could now only hope he would eventually get a GED on his own impetus. As his mother, she knew who he was, his capabilities, and his academic limitations. He could not conform to the school's academic regulations. The principal told him to go and clean out his locker, and Tom left the room. Janet felt sad and disappointed but attempted to understand Tom's decision from his viewpoint.

And at that moment, Tom quit school. On the way home, Janet felt a deep sadness as she traveled those 34 miles. She also chided herself because she knew successful people who never completed high school. Her mind raced as she attempted to strategize on how to capitalize on her son's abilities and make them work for him. Tom never did return to school, even though many of his close friends and his mother encouraged him to do so.

Home for Christmas

Although I felt despondent about Tom leaving school, I aimed to keep joy within the household. Christmas was always a time of cheer, and this year I would enjoy spending the holidays with him.

Excerpt from Janet's Journal

Although this would be the last Christmas that Janet would celebrate with Tom, they created some happy memories. This passage describes the time they spent together.

"Snow was lightly falling, as I drove through the country to pick up Tom at his father's and bring him home for Christmas. I felt excited about seeing Tom and sharing Christmas with him. His brother, Tim, graduated from high school in June 1995 and had enlisted in the Army. Tim could not come home for the holidays. Buying and wrapping gifts for Tom in a way that would disguise the contents had become a tradition, and I delighted once more in the game. He loved to guess, so it proved to be a challenge to outsmart him.

That year I argued with myself about the practicality of putting up a tree and decorating it. Since the boys grew older and lived with their father, they only came in for an overnight on Christmas Eve. After arguing with myself, I decided to put up a Christmas tree.

On the drive to pick up Tom, I felt nostalgic, reminiscing past Christmas celebrations with my boys. We enjoyed the fun, excitement, and wonder that Christmas brings. My mind traveled to past Christmas days when the boys and I would decorate the Christmas tree the day after Thanksgiving and enjoy it for at least a month in anticipation of Christmas. They seemed enchanted by the flashing lights, tinsel, and the ornaments on the tree, checking the homemade special ornaments they previously made in school. We enjoyed Christmas programs on television, listened to Christmas carols, and celebrated the birth of Christ.

I would allow them to open a small gift every night after school starting December 1st until Christmas Day. Opening a small gift helped ease the long wait until Christmas. It may have been batteries for their toys, gum, a candy bar, or other such gifts. Christmas time felt busy, as we looked forward to upcoming festivities at their school and church.

Lately, I found myself grieving and longing for those special moments when the boys were younger. As the boys moved away and matured, Christmas was just not the same. I attempted to capture special times with them as before, but they were different. They were growing up. As I drove along, my reverie was broken as I realized I passed the driveway to Tom's father's home.

As I pulled in the driveway, I beeped the horn and Tom bounded out of the back door bouncing like Tigger in the "Pooh Bear" tales. He anticipated the Christmas holiday. As we traveled back to Niagara Falls, we talked non-stop. On Tom's previous visits, we had the best conversations as Tom would open his heart discussing any major concerns with me or sharing his adventures. This time as we arrived home, Tom's eyes lit up as he saw the Christmas decorations, admired the bright lights on the tree, and looked for the personal tree ornaments he had previously made in school. He folded his six-foot-plus frame on the floor and began sorting through the wrapped gifts under the tree looking for the presents bearing his name. He, of course, tried to guess what was in the packages. His expression of delight and excitement proved to me that the effort of decorating the tree was worth it.

Tom told me he needed to go shopping for a few more presents for Christmas. Tom and I enjoyed shopping together at the mall, as we would go our separate ways, meet at a given place, or sometimes just shop together. We both loved a bargain!! I gave him my Christmas requests which included needle nose pliers, a level, and the video, *Mr. Holland's Opus*. I needed the tools and wanted the video, but most of all, I knew Tom could easily buy them.

As we looked through the stores at the mall for his purchases, he found me and asked me if I would buy him a Nike baseball hat. Tom loved to wear baseball hats. Since the baseball hat cost too much that day, I deliberated. He sensed my hesitation, and once again, "Mr. Persuasion" began to work his magic. Tom would first find a way to rephrase the question—a nice way of trying to convince me. When I would say, "No", and before the third request, he would leave me alone. His quietness did not mean he had placed the request behind him. It was his way of thinking up another strategy to convince me of his need for the object. Tom had a nice way of being, "gently pushy!"

I decided to buy him the hat. After I told him I would buy it for him, he could not contain his excitement and immediately put his hat on his head. His face lit up as he smiled and thanked me for it. I knew I made the right decision!

Christmas Eve afternoon, Tom and his best friend, Craig, hung out in the garage listening to music and wrapping presents. I kept teasing him that I really wanted the video I requested. He sounded convincing as he kept giving me reasons why he could not buy it for me. I almost believed him. As he brought his presents into the house and placed them under the tree, I had an opportunity to closely examine the gifts like an excited child, anticipating the package that resembled a video. It was nowhere to be found!!

We went to church that evening. The church was the natural setting to remember and celebrate the birth of Jesus, sing Christmas carols, and share with others what God had done in our lives. Tom did not mind going to church most of the time and during the busy Christmas season, he willingly accepted the season's special meaning.

As we arrived home, Tom suggested we open a present. I looked for one in the shape of a video but saw none. I was puzzled. *Did he forget to get it for me?* He knew how much I wanted it. Instead, I opened a gift of a telephone (before cell phones!) for the basement. After it was unwrapped, he said, "I know, Mom, you want me to install it??!!!"

"Thank you, Tom, you know how frustrated I get when attempting to install electronics," I replied. Tom chose the present of tools I bought him so he could fix his car. He was excited that he could add them to his existing collection.

We watched the movie *National Lampoon's Christmas Vacation*. Each Christmas, we enjoyed it as we laughed and laughed. "Hey, Ma!!" he said with a straight and convincing look, "when I grow up, I want to be like cousin Eddie."

"No, you don't," I retorted. He always enjoyed getting a reaction from me. He knew how to push my buttons knowing I would not want him to be like cousin Eddie.

On Christmas Day, he awakened before I did. He came into my bedroom, diving onto the other side of the bed. "Mom, get up so we can open up our presents!" he demanded.

"Alright, as long as you have *Mr. Holland's Opus* for me," I teased.

We opened one present at a time. He unwrapped the package containing a striped shirt, then put it on, modeling the Nike hat I bought him the night before. He looked puzzled at the last gift, struggling to guess the contents. Taunting him, I said, "SO, I got you this time, Tom!" I enjoyed stumping him. He tore off the wrapping paper and discovered a gym bag with his initials on it. I had been successful in fooling him! I took a picture of him modeling his new shirt, holding his bag with his initials, and his Nike hat, a picture I hold dear today.

I unwrapped the packages containing the level and the needle nose pliers, which I needed for my tool kit. Finally, he handed me the last box. The box was in the shape of a hexagon. As I unwrapped it, I realized that it was a Domino's pizza box. Opening it, I saw the video taped to the inside bottom of the box! Of course, Tom sat there with an arrogant grin on his face delighting in every moment, knowing he fooled me. I finally admitted to him I did not think he bought me the video!

We called Tim, his brother, in Savannah, and talked with him as he unwrapped his gifts, wishing he could be with us.

We enjoyed Christmas brunch with friends, then I drove Tom back to his father's home. He tried convincing me to let him drive, but the snow was falling fast and accumulating so I decided to drive.

I dropped Tom off at his father's with his Christmas presents and a hug and a kiss!! Unbeknownst to me, it would be our last Christmas together."

Our Last Vacation Together (1997)

Buoyed and revived from the joy of her Christmas memories with Tom, Janet decided to take a bolder step. Weeks after the holiday, she began to plan, looking for a way to be together as a family. As she wrote:

"Early in January, I made plans to fly alone to visit my son, Tim, who lived in Savannah, serving in the Army. I had not seen Tim since he joined the Army one year earlier. During my vacation, I also planned to visit friends in Georgia. I decided to fly to Savannah at the end of February and stay for two weeks. In early February, about two weeks before my flight, I felt this intense urge to take Tom with me. I remembered telling a friend that I did not know what was going to happen, but I felt compelled to be together as a family. Tom seemed frustrated, discouraged, and lacked direction in his life. Nothing seemed to be working out for him. He still did not have a job, continued to drive his car without a license, even though he had been caught once, and been in one accident, plus he showed no desire to return to school. I hoped that spending time with his brother, Tim, would be a source of encouragement for Tom. I also knew they would enjoy each other's company.

The day I checked with the airlines, two weeks before the trip, the rates were high. Our friends, Jim and Gerry, in Georgia were expecting me, but not Tom. I ask them if they would mind if Tom visited as well. Their sincere, gracious hospitality was evident. Jim said, "We would love to have Tom come and spend time with us. I would love to be instrumental in his life as I have been in Tim's life." Jim had been a good role model for my boys, and they admired him. I prayed I would get a good airline rate, and my prayers were answered later in the day when someone had canceled so I bought the airline ticket for a good price! I had met Jim, who served in the Air Force and practiced as a traveling nurse anesthetist, at the hospital where I worked as a nurse in the Recovery Room. I became friends with him and his wife and we loved spending time with them.

Tim graduated from Basic and Advanced training and had been stationed at Hunter Army Airfield in Savannah for the last several months. Tim stayed at the motel with us during our visit to get out of the barracks for a while. Since the boys no longer lived with me, I observed their enjoyment of one another and the reduction of sibling rivalry that normally took place. Their relationship had flourished as they matured.

The next day, Tim showed us around the airfield and the hangar where he worked and introduced us to some of his friends and co-workers. I took pictures of Tim and Tom around the helicopters. Tom seemed interested and with his mechanical ability, and I pondered the possibility of Tom joining the Army when he turned 17. However, I reminded myself the Army required a high school diploma.

That same day, Tim took us flying. Before Tim left home for basic training, he obtained his pilot's license. Due to his Army responsibilities, he did not have a lot of time to practice flying. Since Savannah's weather proved more predictable, he tried to find as much time as possible to practice flying and hoped to gain his instrument rating. I had never flown with Tim piloting the plane before and felt a bit anxious. I trusted him due to his competence in this area and his usual prudent choices.

I sat in the back seat and Tom sat in front. Even though Tim's take-off was smooth, a sudden tinge of nausea hit me as it sometimes happened in smaller airplanes. I braced myself and took deep breaths as we ascended. Once Tim gained the altitude needed and leveled off in the air, my nausea settled down. Tom previously flew with him and enjoyed it. At one point, Tom tempted Tim to take some risks and do some tricks while in the air. Of course, that is all I had to hear, and I spoke up rather quickly!

We flew along the Savannah River and took in the beautiful sights from miles up. We enjoyed the majestic view of the marshes, the lighthouse, Fort Pulaski, and much more. Clouds began to gather after a short time, and Tim returned to the airport since he did not have his instrument rating. His landing was smooth as I sat in the backseat, proud of him. He felt elated to have taken us up, even though I was relieved to be back on land!

The following day, Tom and I traveled three hours to see our friends Jim and Gerry. During our visit with them before bedtime, unbeknownst to me, Tom asked Jim some searching questions about life, the ethics of war, and spiritual decisions. As the conversation continued, I went to bed. As I later learned, their discussions led Tom to ask Jim if he ever signed the back of his driver's license regarding organ donation. Jim replied that he had signed the back of his license. Tom said, "When I get my driver's license, I want to do the same." He went on to say, "If anything ever happens to me, I want to donate my organs so others can live."

Tom never shared this with me. Jim took Tom to the Job Corps the following day. They found out the requirements to enroll, as Jim encouraged Tom to finish his education.

Returning to Savannah a few days later, Tom and I decided to go on a boat ride to see the dolphins. It was a rather balmy day, with clear visibility. As I drove slowly toward Tybee Island, I took in the beauty as Spanish moss hung from the trees almost touching the car as well as the median filled with beautiful magenta azaleas. It was a treat from the grayness of Western New York's sights at this time of year. We crossed the flatlands and bridges on route 80 covering the swampland. During our boat ride, we enjoyed watching the agile dolphins jump up out of the water, an art that seems so simple, yet so characteristic of them. Tom possessed an insatiable enthusiasm to learn new things and he found them fascinating as he continued to attempt to take pictures of them. Although the dolphins were too fast to properly photograph, he finally captured a picture of one. At the end of the boat ride, the guide gave everyone a postcard of a dolphin, recognizing the difficulty of photographing them.

Tom and I traveled further down Tybee Island to visit Fort Pulaski. As we entered, you would have thought Tom was the guide. Tom explained the engineering of the fort, even though he had never been there before. He was always interested in how things worked.

We enjoyed spending several hours there, taking in the sights. I remember capturing a particular picture of Tom standing on the turret looking out into the distance. Even though Tom was funny, impulsive, and could drive you crazy with his endless energy and activity, he had his serious moments. Someplace within my soul, I knew even though he could not conform to the demands of school, in his own way, he developed his own intelligence. I felt proud of what he could articulate with such naturalness and logic. That evening Tim joined us as we ate at a restaurant on Tybee Island.

The following day we packed our things, hugged each other, and said our goodbyes. I will never forget where we stood together one last time as a family, not knowing what was ahead. We drove to the airport and returned to Western New York.

After we returned from vacation, Tom returned to his father's home. He felt refreshed and excited. I hoped Tom's visit to the Job Corps in Georgia might spur his interest and motivate him to return to school. I explored the Job Corps in Niagara Falls and spoke with the local guidance counselors and the principal in charge of the GED program in the city. I was informed that Tom could not enroll in the GED program until he was 17 years old, which would be on August 19th, his birthday. They further explained an interview with Tom would be necessary to secure his cooperation and commitment to the program. Strict rules regarding attendance and homework would be expected. I hoped by August he might be willing to consider these options. However, I recognized that I showed more interest in the Niagara Falls GED program than he did at this time."

Mother's Day Surprise (May 1997)

The day before Mother's Day, Tom drove in and spent some time with his friends. He called me and invited me for a Mother's Day dinner. I felt puzzled at first since he usually bought me a hanging pot of flowers. He drove to my house, and we headed to Applebee's, one of our favorite restaurants. Tom enjoyed driving my Nissan Stanza, and I noticed he seemed so confident and secure as he drove; although when he was tempted to speed, I would quickly put an end to it.

After we parked and prepared to exit the car, Tom requested I reach under the seat. There was a Mother's Day card for me. The front of the card showed a woman sitting on a beach with a drink in her hand, reading a book. Tom signed it – "Love, Tom," and I thanked him. It was special, and I still hold it dear today.

Due to the Mother's Day holiday, the restaurant was crowded that night, but we talked through our meal nonstop. Our waiter was busy as we were ready to leave, but I noticed that Tom gave the money for our bill to another waiter. As we were driving home, Tom told me that he did not tip our waiter because he did not have enough money!! I said I would have helped him, but Tom figured the waiter probably received a lot of tips that night because they were busy!!! I further told him the next time to ask me for the money.

I could not have imagined at that moment that this would be our last Mother's Day together.

Another Visit Home - June 1997

Still concerned about Tom's driving without a license, I offered to enroll him in driving school and pay for lessons if he would come to Niagara Falls for a few weeks. He had been stopped twice by the police while driving without a license and had been in two accidents, fortunately without injury. I knew Tom was frustrated and discouraged.

Tom made his own arrangements for lessons with the driving school in Niagara Falls. After his first lesson, he shared his excitement with me stating his female teacher complimented him on his driving and told him it would not take long to complete the program and pass the New York state driving test. The road test was scheduled for June 19th. He felt encouraged, to say the least.

During those three weeks, I let Tom drive around town with me. He seemed secure when I was in the car with him, as I gave him limits when he needed them. With his increased self-confidence, he decided to apply for several jobs around town.

One employer requested that Tom come in and assist him with some office duties. Tom took care of some menial tasks for him but was excited about the possibility of installing car radios, as he had for others. The employer was not ready yet for him to do that and stated he would call him in the future. It was a start. Tom would need to be persistent about getting a job, as no other employers had made contact. At 16 and a high school dropout, I was hopeful of finding an employer who would be willing to hire him.

When Tom visited, he went to church with me. On Sunday, June 1st, Tom sat in church more intent on receiving the message and applying it to his life. The minister spoke on "Wanted–A Man." The sermon focused on the healing of the crippled man who went to Bethsaida, (a house of mercy) which was the right place to be met by the right person who could heal him of his infirmity of 38 years. Christ showed compassion to the man, as the crippled man demonstrated faith by rising from his bed so he could be healed. The minister focused on returning to the Right Person, the Person of Christ, not to an ordinance or a ritual, to meet his needs and then to follow Christ's example of compassion. After the sermon, Tom told the minister he enjoyed the sermon. It touched his heart. To my knowledge, he had never been so attentive nor had he ever complimented the minister after church. As we traveled home, he stated, "Mom, I needed that message today."

We relished the wonderful talks we had during those three weeks. Among the conversations included his statement of caring for me when I became older. We had never discussed this before, so his serious tone of voice surprised me. "Mom, when you get older, I cannot deal with caring for you, so I am planning on putting you in a nursing home!"

I laughed out loud, thinking this discussion was a bit premature since I was 47 years old. I replied, "Tom, you do not need to worry about that because in our family people die suddenly, and it is usually from heart problems." Focusing again on obtaining a GED, I said, "Tom, I know one of these days you will get a GED, and if I am no longer alive, I just ask that you put a copy of the diploma on my gravestone."

He replied, "Whatever you do, do not give up on me!"

I answered, "I will not give up on you! I want the best for you."

Whenever Tom visited, he would talk nonstop about multiple areas of concern in his everyday life and relationships. I listened, provided direction, tried to remain positive, and continued to pray with him.

That June, my tenant's five-year-old son graduated from kindergarten. They lived at one of my apartments on the same property as me. His mother invited us to attend a small party after his graduation. I had a previous engagement, so Tom attended the party on his own.

When I returned, shortly after 9:00 p.m., Tom followed me through the house. In an energetic, but low-toned voice, he said, "Mom, I'm glad I attended his party!"

Curiously, I asked, "Why?"

He said, "Mom, guess who didn't come?" With a hurt and disappointed look on his face and tears in his eyes, his voice cracked as he stumbled out the answer to his own question. "His dad," he said with tears in his eyes. I was glad I could be there for him."

"I am sure it meant a lot to him for you to be there."

"Mom, we have to get him a present."

I answered. "I know. I just have not had a chance yet."

Tom's next response stunned me. "I want to buy him something with my money." My son's sensitivity touched my heart.

"Tom, you are so gracious and giving."

The next day, we stopped at McDonald's after church and Tom purchased a gift certificate, which he later gave to the young lad.

Tom loved to socialize, and whenever he came to visit, he enjoyed talking with friends in the neighborhood. My curfew for him was 10:00 p.m. and most of the time he conformed. When he returned, I would usually be reading in my bed as he would plop himself on the other side of the bed and tell me about his adventures. After he would get ready for bed, Tom would summon me to his room and ask me to pray for him before he settled down for slumber. I loved and cherished our conversations and those special moments.

One night in particular sticks out in my mind. Tom felt discouraged and frustrated. He did not desire to move back with me and perhaps he could not, nor did he want to stay with his father. He had been free for too long. Tom's father and I represented different parenting styles. I attempted to hold my children accountable for their behavior and had a few rules. Like most adolescents, he challenged my rules.

I recall looking at him one night very seriously and saying "Tom, God has a purpose for you." His doubtful expression revealed he was not quite convinced. I told him finding his purpose was the most difficult part, but God would reveal it to him. I went on to say, "God gave you wonderful abilities, and the important thing is to let God use them. You are kind, sensitive, gracious, generous, sociable, witty, a hard worker, easygoing, business-minded, and mechanical." I temporarily ran out of adjectives, but throughout my monologue I observed the tension dissipating from his body. He relaxed and his countenance demonstrated a look of hope. We prayed together that night asking God to show Tom the purpose for his life.

On June 16th, I returned home later than usual but had left a message on my answering machine to inform Tom. When I arrived home after 10:00, Tom was not there but he had left a message on the answering machine indicating that he was at a neighbor's house to discuss employment and would be home soon.

I waited and waited, but Tom did not arrive. At about midnight on that June evening, I walked down the street to my neighbor's house and knocked on the door since they were still awake. He and his wife both indicated they had not seen Tom the entire evening.

Now I was concerned, upset, and angry because Tom lied to me and did not contact me. I prayed a lot and tried to calm myself down, imagining all kinds of terrible things that could have happened. In a fit of hysteria, I drove my car around several blocks, searching for my son, as well as contacting his friends, who had not been in touch with him. Tom was nowhere in sight. Exasperated, I returned home and went to bed, filled with angst.

At 1:30 a.m. Tom came into the house and went to bed as if nothing had happened. I felt furious but decided to wait until the next day to discuss this with him. I knew I needed to hold him accountable for lying to me, staying out over three hours past his curfew, and not contacting me. I later explained to him my continual expectation of following my few rules when he visited me. I shared my concern for his safety and felt deeply disappointed that he failed to contact me to update his status or request permission to stay out later.

I told him I felt a consequence was in order and canceled his driving test. I informed him he could take it on a later date—his birthday on August 19th. Tom felt angry, hurt, and livid as he explained this to his father on the phone. He then and there decided to return to his father's home as I packed his belongings. Tom requested his friend's mother drive him. I started to cry but let him know a consequence was necessary, and I wanted him to succeed.

He answered in an adamant manner, "Success is getting my license!" Our conversation ended as I told Tom I loved him and that he would be able to test later. Without comment, he left to return to his father's home.

What I learned later from his friends was that keeping early morning hours was his practice, which I was unaware of. Tom later explained to me that he was visiting a 31-year-old single mother of two boys who lived in an apartment across the street. Then I asked why he failed to contact me. I also questioned why this single mother allowed him to be there until 1:30 a.m. Privately, I wondered why she did not inquire as to whether his mother knew where he was.

2

A Fatal Foreshadowing

Janet's Journal Continued - July 1997

"I remember feeling intensely sad for Tom after he left that day. Shortly after he left, I felt desperate, humanly powerless, and fell on my knees, weeping in God's presence. As a mother, I knew his abilities and weaknesses, but most of all, his potential. I felt utterly frustrated and cried out to God in despair, reminding Him of my efforts to help Tom. Maintaining my faith through it all, I tried everything in my power to provide the guiding hand he needed to obtain a high school diploma, a job, and the willingness to develop his potential with God's help. If only he returned to live with me. Yet, at this time, my faith was faltering, and I could think of nothing else to do for my son but continue to pray. I felt powerless to change his mind to return to Niagara Falls to live with me. All I could do was turn him over to God.

In my mind, I thought of the illustration in Barbara Johnson's self-titled book, *The Best of Barbara Johnson, Splashes of Joy in the Cesspools of Life,* Copyright 1992, Inspirational Press NY. It was a picture of stairs with Jesus sitting at the top in a chair, a reference to handing your children to the Lord. Even though I played it through my mind many times before, I visually walked Tom up the stairs in my arms and handed him to God one last time, saying "Lord, again, I give him to you. I submit to your will. Please give me wisdom for the days ahead, and if there is anything else you want me to do, please let me know." I thanked God for giving Tom to me. Then I visually walked back down the stairs, looking back with Tom safely in the loving arms of Jesus.

However, during the prayer, I visualized three doors on earth closing for Tom. They were the doors of work, his driver's license opportunity, and his education. As I arose from my knees, I felt this false sense of peace; but it was overshadowed by a pending sense of doom for Tom. Something bad was going to happen to him, but I did not know what it was. Consciously, I could not even fathom that it might be death. Still, for the next six weeks, I carried around this heavy feeling of underlying sadness, none of which could be explained with reason. Later, I recognized I was prematurely grieving over Tom's anticipatory death.

I did not want to think about it, feeling paralyzed. So I continued to pray, read the Bible for comfort and escaped into reading novels. As soon as I finished one book, I would immediately start another to distract my mind. My favorite spot to read was near the beautiful Niagara River. The last novel I read was called *Family Blessings*, a book about a 46-year-old mother who lost her 25-year-old son in a motorcycle accident. I completed this book the day before Tom died.

I did not know the single mom across the street, so at one point during this six-week period, I told my tenant about the incident and expressed my concern that she would allow him to stay until 1:30 a.m. Somehow, the word got back to her, and she called me on June 23rd. Her apologetic voice spoke volumes. She told me she encouraged Tom to contact me at 10:00 p.m., but he ignored her request. She further informed me that she invited Tom to attend her sons' Little League games with them earlier that evening, adding, "My boys really like Tom."

When they returned to her home, Tom fixed some things around her apartment. The boys did not go to bed until 11:30 p.m. She complained to Tom about her attempt to try being both mom and dad, being a single mom. "I was surprised with Tom's response," she said.

He said to her, "Do not try to be a dad, just be a mom!" Wise words!

She noted, "I stopped in my tracks and suddenly felt better." As it turned out, they watched a video until 1:30 a.m., and then Tom left to return home."

Calling Tom

It was a week before I called Tom. I thought it would give both of us time to regroup before reconnecting. I told him of my conversation with the single mom and that she apologized to me. He seemed defensive and distant but reluctantly discussed the incident. Tom further shared some ideas for possible future plans exploring options for his life. He sounded like a ship without a rudder. Most of the time, I did not know what to believe. In fact, a few weeks before he died, he called his friend who lived down the street and told him he planned to move in with a friend, and it would be the last time he would be talking to him. His friend felt distressed over this and later said, "It was as if Tom was saying goodbye." Perhaps he was.

Fourth of July - 1997

Tom loved the July 4th holiday. Each year he would purchase firecrackers in Ohio or Pennsylvania. Sometimes he would sell them to others, make a few bucks, and shoot off the rest of them, expressing his entrepreneurial ability. When he was younger, as a family we would attend fireworks shows which he loved. Now an adolescent, he preferred to spend time with friends during the Fourth of July. After arriving at his friend Craig's home, he called to inform me that he would come and visit me the following day.

His Last Visit - July 5

The next afternoon, he drove his car to my house, and I immediately sensed his high anxiety due to his fear of getting caught driving without a license. He felt proud of his car, enjoyed fixing it up, putting in speakers, and a stereo with a CD player. In an animated voice, he said, "Mom, I want you to drive my car." I had not driven a standard car in some time but decided to try it if only to share Tom's excitement of showing the car to me.

I drove around the block with some irregularity as we laughed about my challenge with driving a stick shift. Tom was delighted! As we returned to the house, Tom stayed for about 15 minutes. He did not come into the house but did walk up the driveway with me. As I walked back down the driveway with him, Tom shared a disturbing revelation.

"My father and I are going to a family reunion in Ohio and need to take two cars because we are bringing a lot of beer. I will be driving one of the cars."

I felt befuddled and could only muster up a "Wow," before asking what seemed like an obvious question. "Why can't you buy beer in Ohio?" I remember feeling both surprised and saddened at the same time.

But Tom's next question floored me. "You are not going to turn us into the sheriff, are you?"

I was taken aback. Did he want me to? Why did he even mention it? I was still thinking about it as he gave me a hug and a kiss and then drove away—for the last time ever from my home.

Tom's Last Two Weeks

About two weeks before his death, I was working in the kitchen on a Saturday morning. Unexpectedly, the following thought came into my mind, "What would you do if Tom died?" It was not a morbid thought, although I did entertain it, unlike other times when rare thoughts of my children dying would be too painful to bear and I would dismiss them. However, today it seemed different.

I immediately began to plan for his funeral. I reviewed who and what would console me. I would choose Pastor Marvin Engle to perform the funeral service because he had such a profound spiritual influence on my life and could comfort me through the Scriptures. He performed my father's funeral in 1975, which my dad had requested.

Because I find Christian music comforting, I chose Vicki, a beautiful soloist, knowing her God-given talent and passion for singing would bring me solace. She later reminded me through her voice that God is sufficient to meet my needs and is always there for me.

Even at this point, I still had not fully comprehended that Tom's death was imminent. I still had this feeling of impending doom, although I had not yet placed all the pieces of the puzzle together. It was not until I spoke with a friend on the day of Tom's death that she helped me put it all in perspective, and then I cried. I saw it unfold in front of me as to how God prepared me for Tom's homegoing.

Our Last Meal Together - July 24, 1997

On Thursday, July 24th, I went to the dentist in Lockport. (I would learn later that on July 31st, just one week later, my dentist would also lose his 13-year-old son in a bicycle accident while on vacation—just two days before Tom died.) Following my dental appointment, I visited an ex-tenant of mine who recently gave birth to their first son. Being unable to attend her baby shower, I visited with her and brought a present for her son. It was enjoyable to hold him as she shared her excitement about his birth.

Teresa lived in an apartment at my house for five years, and she inquired about my boys. My sons used to care for and play with her dog. Our conversation turned toward my graver concern for Tom, confiding in her that I felt this impending doom about him. Her tone was serious and heartfelt as she later described what I projected to her.

Leaving her home, I drove to pick up Tom by 3:00 p.m., as we previously discussed, to spend time with him. I allowed him to drive, which always excited him. He drove me around a familiar small lakeside community, acted as a tour guide, and then drove to a restaurant he and his dad, grandfather, and brother previously frequented. The boys spent many happy times sailing with their grandfather and their dad. We sat in the corner, next to the water, and talked non-stop.

"Tom, do you miss sailing?" I asked. His countenance suddenly changed into disappointment and hurt.

He then replied, "Mom, do you see that boat?" pointing to one tied in the harbor.

Saying that I did, he responded, "It's Grampa's boat."

"How do you know?"

He said, "Because I know." I believed he did. (Tom's father later told me that he had recently asked for his grandfather and said he wanted him back.) His grandfather used to take him sailing and died in 1987 when Tom was just seven years old.

I let Tom drive back to his father's and he told me he had a tarp on the front end of his car because he had been in an accident. After we pulled into the driveway, I got out and checked out his car. He had not been in an accident. I gave him a hug and got back into the car. Law enforcement knew his car so he had placed a tarp on it.

Tom revealed to me that he had again been pulled over by police and received a ticket for impersonation, using his brother's ID, and driving without a license. I remember exactly where Tom was standing as he shared this with me. He felt upset again that he was caught driving without a license and was scheduled to attend court on his birthday, August 19th, where they would consider suspending his driving permit. Following his court date, he planned to move to Ohio. It seemed he was grasping at straws and did not know what to do next.

I then said to him, "Tom, you are not making wise decisions and I'm worried about your life and your future. Please, please, Tom, I beg of you to return home!!!"

After listening to Tom for a while, I told him I loved him, would continue to pray for him, and then drove away with my faith faltering. That would be the last time I would ever see him alive.

Last Conversation with Tom - Tuesday, July 29, 1997 - 10:00 p.m.

I called Tom to talk with him, as I did a few times during the week, to see how he was doing. He explained some grandiose plans and seemed to be rudderless. He still could not find a job and made it clear that he did not want to stay with me or his father. He begged to stay with friends, but they said no. Then he wrote to his cousin to inquire if he could move in with him.

Our conversation was short. Neither of us had much to say.

However, since he was discussing some big ideas he had, I prefaced my comments by saying, "Tell me what's REALLY going on." He went on to reply that he and his friends had gone to a park and enjoyed themselves.

After he shared his adventures, I ended the conversation with "I have to go now, but I love you."

He retorted, "I love you, too, Mom."

That was the last time I would hear those words from him. I hold them close to my heart; a memory I will always savor.

God lent Tom to us for 16 years, 349 days, and 20 hours.

Hartland Road

Rural northwestern New York is a grid of two-lane roads marking boundaries of farmers' fields. Most north-south roads run straight as a plumbline and stutter their comments down the centers with white broken lines for passing. Occasionally, a solid white line warns of a rise in the road.

Hartland Road cuts through dairy pastures, growing feed, and some fruit farms from its northern point on Lake Road to its southern end on Route 31.

This north-south road is a driver's paradise. On a hot summer night, this is a great run for a cool ride at a "good speed." Junctions with east-west roads are well lit, so the one or two vehicles out at 10:00 p.m. can see approaching traffic at the crossroads.

3

A Parent's Worst Nightmare

On a warm summer night on August 2, 1997, I had just hung up the telephone after finishing a conversation with a friend just before 11:00 p.m. I walked toward my bedroom to get ready for bed when my phone rang.

It was Tom's father telling me Tom had been in an accident and the ambulance had taken him to a country hospital nearby. His father was waiting for the helicopter to arrive at the small hospital to transport Tom to Erie County Medical Center (ECMC)—the trauma center in Western New York.

My first question was simple. "How did the accident happen?" My second was more poignant and telling. "Was Tom in a car, walking, or riding with someone else?"

His dad hesitated for what seemed like minutes and then responded by telling me Tom was on his motorcycle and had taken a ride up the road. Because Tom did not return right away, he set out to find him. As he drove up the road, he saw flashing red lights and an ambulance as this sickening feeling overcame him, wondering if Tom was involved.

As his father approached, he found Tom lying in the road, unresponsive, in awful shape, with blood coming out of his ears. He knelt beside Tom, assuring him help was on the way.

He then told me Tom moved his extremities. Hearing that, I felt somewhat better, consoling myself that perhaps his condition was serious but not critical.

His dad was never fond of medical jargon, and knowing how upset anyone would be in finding their child in a perilous condition, I was not sure of the severity of the injuries. I told him I would meet them at ECMC.

I tried not to panic or expect the worst before hearing an update from a doctor. I made several phone calls to my friends and family, sharing the awful news, and asking them to pray. They all said they would. I then called my nurse friend Judy, who worked at the local hospital in the ER. She said she would take me to ECMC. As we drove there, I honestly did not know what to expect but prayed silently as I hoped for the best.

After we arrived at about 12:30 a.m., I introduced myself to the emergency room staff. They stated the physician would talk with us soon. One of the emergency medical technicians (EMT) had driven Tom's father to ECMC and we were introduced. The EMT seemed anxious to go home since he checked with me to make sure his father had a ride home. Since our arrival the EMT looked so-o-o-o sad. In retrospect, although it did not occur to me at the time, after assessing Tom at the accident scene, he was classified as a 3 on the Glasgow scale. This EMT already knew Tom was not going to make it. I, of course, was unaware.

The Glasgow Coma Scale (GCS) is a measure to assess neurological function. The scoring range is 3-15, and the total is based on three categories that are graded 1-5. The minimum score is a 3 which indicates a deep coma or a brain-dead state. The maximum is 15 which indicates a fully awake patient. (The original maximum was 14, but the score has since been modified).

We were not sure of the details of the accident at that time. A witness later reported that Tom drove in the proper lane of the road, with his helmet on, traveling slowly when a 19-year-old girl, speeding because she was late picking up her mother, did not see Tom and hit him from behind. He was ejected from the motorcycle and catapulted backward, hitting her windshield and knocking him unconscious. His helmet flew off as Tom rolled over her car and landed in the middle of the road—178 feet from the point of impact on his head. It seemed like an eternity before the physician called us in to give us a report of Tom's condition. I had been in the waiting room with Judy while Tom's father waited outside with the parents of the girl that hit Tom and their neighbors who he knew. The girl had also been flown to the hospital suffering minor injuries. As I walked out of the emergency room to tell Tom's dad that the physician wanted to speak with us, he introduced the girl's parents and their neighbors to me.

We went into a small room near the emergency room where Tom's neurosurgeon gave us the grave news of Tom's poor prognosis. After viewing the CT-Scans, he described the extensive head trauma and explained Tom's brain would swell and eventually herniate, which is always fatal.

We were offered two bleak options. Either we could allow Tom to die on life support or opt for surgery to relieve the intracranial pressure. The neurosurgeon further revealed that even if surgery was successful, Tom only had a 5% chance of survival, would remain in a vegetative state, and never talk again.

During this brief process of communication from the neurosurgeon, the information came faster than my ability to process it or even believe it. I cannot describe the incredible pain. No news could have hurt me more than to learn one of my children was dying. It felt like someone stabbing me in the heart and taking my breath away at the same time! To try and make my mind comprehend that my precious son lay there dying did not seem possible, and I refused to believe it. My thoughts traveled to my work as a nurse caring for patients in vegetative states, knowing it was merely an existence, not a life. I knew that even though I could pray for a miracle for Tom to remain alive, and if God willed it, the intensity of brain damage would preclude a quality of life. I knew Tom would not be Tom if he could not talk.

I felt powerless, knowing I could not nurture the bruise away! Reflecting on the physician's words and knowing the severity of injuries, I knew life was over for Tom. Hearing those words, I prayed, "Lord, please take him quickly." It was a parent's worst nightmare!

As the neurosurgeon turned around and walked toward the door, he said, "You may want to consider organ donation." As soon as I heard "organ donation," the stark reality hit me again—my son was going to die! I knew no physician would ever mention organ donation unless recovery was impossible. Because I was in shock, I would not have thought about asking the neurosurgeon about organ donation, so I was glad he brought it up.

However, I continued to cling to the 5% hope, praying that surgery would tell another story. Being a nurse, I told myself that perhaps when they operated, it might not be as bad as he described. Emotionally, I was not yet ready to relinquish Tom.

"Can we see Tom?" I asked the neurosurgeon.

"An MRI is being taken and when completed, you can see him."

Rationalizing in my mind, I told myself, "Maybe the Magnetic Resonance Imaging (MRI) will be wrong. Maybe they will read the wrong MRI, or perhaps God could perform a miracle." We hoped against hope the situation would change for the better and were unwilling to let go of the 5% hope. (An MRI is a medical imaging technique using a magnetic field and computer-generated radio waves to create a detailed image of the organs/tissues in your body. It serves as a diagnosing technique for diseases or injury and can also monitor treatment.)

His father and I looked at each other and knew organ donation would be a certainty. I had several thoughts at the time. Even though Tom and I never broached the subject, I knew my son was a giving person and would want to give life to others. That is who he was. He loved life and he loved people! I recall thinking, *Since death is out of my hands, I do have a choice about life for others.* Deciding to donate Tom's organs, bones, and tissues seemed like the obvious and logical decision to make.

Making that decision brought me solace, knowing others would live during the darkest night of my life. Because I believed that Tom's body was a house for his soul, I knew at the time of death, he would no longer need his body. So why not help others? I had confidence Tom would be pleased with that decision, as well.

We were unaware at that time that five months earlier, as was previously stated, he discussed this with Jim in Georgia. Tom stated that if anything happened to him, he would want to donate his organs to help others. I also knew in the back of my mind that at one future point I would want to correspond with, if not actually meet, some of Tom's recipients.

But for now, my most immediate focus remained on trying to believe Tom's death was imminent. I felt utterly devastated and numb with the shocking news of Tom's poor prognosis. I stated to Tom's father, "I only know of one thing to do, and that is to pray. Do you mind if I pray?"

He said "No." I took his hand and thanked God for the years we had with Tom and asked Him for wisdom and strength in the days ahead.

I left the little room and returned to the waiting area to share this news with my friend Judy. I fell into her arms crying and told her Tom was not going to live. I was glad she was there. At the same time, Tom's father returned to his spot just outside the waiting room as the girl's parents and neighbors asked about Tom's condition. Tim told them, "They are waiting for Tom to die!"

A few minutes later, the staff informed us we could see Tom. He lay on the stretcher, head bandaged, on the respirator, with intravenous tubes attached to him and an obvious indentation to his right temple area. I knew he had a cranial fracture. Knowing that hearing is the last sense to leave a dying person, I took his hand and talked to him. I told him how sorry I was that this happened to him. I told him over and over how much I loved him. I reassured Tom he would soon be safe in the arms of God in Heaven.

Our Last Human Hope

Even though I knew Tom's chance of survival was nil, I felt it was too soon to give up hope. Surgery would be our last hope, and I wanted to wait until it was over before resigning myself to the inevitable.

How could I call Tim, his brother? They had grown up together, played together, ate together, and fought together. He would now be the only child. If ever there was a time that I wished I had more children, it was then!

I could not bring myself to call Tim yet. Looking back, I procrastinated, hoping post-operatively that the neurosurgeon would give us a better story than he had initially. Knowing Tom was going to die was difficult enough for me to believe. Sharing this with Tim, his only brother and sibling, was painful to think about, much less convey. I struggled with telling Tim about his brother, knowing I could not be present with him to share the news. Yet, I needed to contact him. I wanted to receive the final report following surgery in the hopes of giving Tim better news.

As the medical staff prepared Tom for surgery, I contacted other family members and friends at 3:00 a.m., leaving messages and talking with others. I also called my minister and told him that Tom was at ECMC and was not expected to live. He stated he would come to the hospital. The prayer chain at our church was initiated. I also encouraged Tom's father to call his family, since he was pacing up and down the hall and needed support. We moved from the emergency room waiting area to the surgical waiting room.

Friends and relatives started arriving shortly thereafter. I felt paralyzed, still stunned by the news, as I felt frozen inside like a block of ice. At the same time as surgery was being performed on Tom, a different surgical doctor performed an operation on another injured motorcyclist who had sustained a head trauma. Their family waited as well in the same room as us. A few hours later, their anesthesiologist came out and talked with them. It seemed this son and brother would live.

The anesthesiologist must have sensed I was listening because he looked at me and said something to the point of, "Your son will not be as fortunate." I felt this pain cut into my heart. I did not want to hear that! All my hopes were vanishing. Why did he have to say that to me?????

My minister and his wife arrived about 4:30 a.m., hugged me, and said prayers with us. Feeling emotionally and mentally overwhelmed by information, words from others seemed inconsequential. However, I appreciated the presence of people as I sat in silence trying to absorb it all while fighting back the reality and resisting tears.

At about 7:30 a.m., the neurosurgeon came out of surgery. He told us, "The medical team may need to perform a tracheotomy on Tom because the endotracheal tube is not staying in place." We discussed this for a while, and then the neurosurgeon said, "Tom's injuries were even worse than we expected. I was able to remove the damaged cranial tissue. The only reason I could not pronounce him dead was that he still has minimal breathing but not enough to sustain life, thus, the respirator. The surgery was performed without anesthesia and, as you know, Tom sustained a cranial fracture." He added, "We'll place him in the Trauma Intensive Care Unit (TICU) until the brain swells enough to herniate the brainstem and obliterate the breathing and cardiac function. The medical staff will perform frequent breathing tests as he declines and will continue to assess his deteriorating condition."

The 5% hope I tenaciously clung to disappeared. All human hope was gone. From the beginning, Tom never responded and ranked low on the neurological scale. I intellectually knew with the amount of injury to Tom's brain his death would be a mercy of God. But emotionally, I was not ready to believe it.

The realization hit me—I must let Tom go.

But how do you let go of your precious child? It was now a waiting game until Tom's spontaneous breathing ended with impending brain herniation, and then he would be pronounced dead.

I felt thankful that Tom was not suffering and that he would soon be ushered into the presence of a loving God. Perhaps the angels were preparing to take him in Heaven, and he would soon meet my mom, dad, and his other grandfather. It brought me a great sense of peace knowing Tom believed in Christ at nine years old, but it was too soon to grasp he would no longer be with us on Earth.

Procrastinating too long already, I finally suggested to Tom's father that we call Tim, who was still serving in the Army and based in Savannah, Georgia. Upon answering the phone, his dad tearfully told him about the events of the night. Tim then requested to talk with me. I repeated the story and apologized for giving him such horrible news about Tom. He, too, felt upset trying to take it all in. I was heartbroken that I could not be with him. Tim and Tom grew up together and shared life together until 18 months ago when Tim enlisted in the military. I felt worse for him than I did myself. He said, "I will stay in touch and make plane reservations to come home."

That day, the headline in the local newspaper read:

Motorcyclist is Critical After Being Struck by Car

My Baby is Dying - August 3, 1997

After I saw Tom again in the TICU, hooked up to the respirator and other supportive devices, I decided to return home. It was 9:00 a.m. on Sunday morning, August 3rd. The minister offered to drive me before he began his church duties. As we rode along, he said, "When I return to church this morning, others will be asking how you are doing. What should I tell them?"

I stated, "I am in shock right now but feel assured that I will be alright with God's help and the prayers of others. However, I have never traveled this road before."

When I arrived home, I contacted other friends and relatives to share the sad news. I called Tom's best friend, Craig, and left a message on his parents' phone requesting a return phone call as soon as possible. I did not want Craig to find out without his parents' present. Tom and Craig enjoyed their friendship for ten years. Tom spent a lot of time at their home, as well.

Craig's dad returned the phone call, and I related the tragic events of the previous night. He was upset, as well, later explaining it to his family. They, too, struggled to believe it. Now Craig was losing his best friend.

Later that afternoon, Nancy, Craig's mother, and I traveled together to the hospital. She wanted to see Tom. As we entered the TICU, I became very clinical, having worked in the Intensive Care Unit earlier in my career. I asked the nurse for updates on Tom's vital signs and intracranial pressure (ICP). Although Tom's vital signs were stable, his ICP was 65-100. The ICP measures the pressure within the head following a severe head injury. The normal ICP is 10-20. Tom's condition was critical. God had taken Tom out of our hands. There were no decisions to make. It became a waiting game!

I held Tom's hand and talked to him. I longed to feel, to cry, but I could not because I was numb. Nancy cried for me as she stood over his bed and wept. Tom looked like he was sleeping. As the harsh cruel reality slowly penetrated my heart and mind, I prayed that Tom would stay alive until his brother arrived.

Nancy and I later picked up Tim at the airport about 7:00 p.m. As Tim entered the terminal, we hugged each other and returned to the hospital. He embraced his father and then he and I went in to see Tom. I felt bad that Tim was faced with his brother's imminent death. He stood over his bed and cried, saying, "I'm sorry for all those things I said about you!"

The neurosurgeon summoned the three of us to a private room to give us an update on Tom's condition. As we sat down, he said, "Tom has the hiccups!"

Grabbing urgently and desperately for anything that might be a sign of hope, I abruptly asked, "Is that a good sign?"

The neurosurgeon further explained, "This is brainstem activity, and even though the breathing tests are within normal limits now, they are decreasing."

My son asked in a rather desperate tone of voice, "Isn't there *anything* else you can do?"

The neurosurgeon replied, "Your brother is out of my hands. He is now in God's hands." Penetrating and agonizing silence filled the room. They were words we did not want to hear as we were continually reminded that Tom was dying. His father and I posed rhetorical questions. "Who would think Tom would die before us? Whoever considers burying your child before yourself?" It all seemed too much to comprehend. Changing directions, we began discussing funeral plans.

Brain death occurs when blood and oxygen cannot flow to the brain. The person's heart is still beating and providing blood and oxygen to the rest of the body because they are on a ventilator. After a severe brain injury, the brain swells, compressing the vascular system and denying any access to oxygen. The swollen brain has no place to go and eventually herniates through the area of the brainstem which controls respiration and heart function. The staff performs breathing tests periodically to assess brain function. The patient is taken off the respirator and observed for any spontaneous breathing. Once the carbon dioxide builds up in the circulation, the brainstem, under healthy situations, involuntarily initiates a breath. If there is no involuntary breath, the brain has herniated, the brainstem is non-functioning, and brain death occurs. The requirement in the state of New York in 1997 required two physicians to collaborate and agree together that brain death has occurred.

During the evening at the hospital, my sisters and brothers, who lived out of the area, tried to fathom the unbelievable and the inevitable as they attempted to console me. Friends sat in the waiting room offering prayers and support. Finally, at 10:00 p.m. I decided to go home and attempt to get some sleep. I had been up for 44 hours. Tim said, "I want to spend the night with Tom." His paternal grandmother also planned on staying, so feeling confident of her presence, I left.

As I entered my home, my neighbors had delivered breakfast food for the next day. It was a welcome sight. The phone calls did not stop. I tried to physically regroup so I could get some sleep as I knew I would need as much physical rest as possible to get through the coming days. I knew since Tom would not be responding and his life nearing the end, I would attempt to get a good night's sleep as my thoughts forged ahead to funeral preparations.

After waking up the next day, I stayed in contact with the staff of TICU. I started planning the funeral service and contacted those individuals who would participate. Later that day, I spoke with the TICU nurse around 2:00 p.m., who reported a breathing test had been performed and another breathing test would be performed much later. So even though I was busy making funeral plans, I knew I had time to return before Tom was pronounced dead.

Due to multiple interruptions, my sister and I left my home later than planned, became lost en route, and parked in the wrong parking area. Tom's father had been attempting to contact me unsuccessfully to inform us that Tom had been pronounced brain dead at 4:03 p.m. following the second breathing test. (This was before cell phones!) As my sister and I arrived, we were still unaware that Tom had been pronounced dead. As we entered the hallway to the TICU, we were welcomed by anxious relatives, friends, and the minister. Tom's father was extremely relieved to see me and sadly broke the news of Tom's pronouncement of death. We then answered questions, signed consents for organ donation, as well as talked with the minister about the funeral service.

How can a mother fathom that her son is dead??? He still looked alive as I entered his room to say goodbye as the sounds of the respirator kept his chest rising and falling. His skin was pink in color, and he was warm to touch, but I cognitively knew he was brain dead. I put my arms around him one last time amidst the tubes and respirator. I said, "Tom, I love you and am glad God chose me to be your mother," as I started to cry. "I will miss you A LOT!" I consoled myself by knowing he was safe, alive in Heaven, his death a mercy of God, and I would see him again. I could never wish him back in his present physical state. I struggled with believing it and knowing he would no longer be with us on Earth, which was heart-wrenching.

The next day as I awoke, I lay there trying to believe the unbelievable. I wrestled between not accepting it and compelling my mind to assimilate its truth as I repeated, "Tom is dead! Tom is dead!." I tried to force the appalling reality in the hope of allowing it to penetrate as tears ran down my face. My heart literally hurt. It was all too much to bear. On that day, August 5th, the paper read: "Motorcyclist dies of injuries." It did not, however, mention that lives were saved due to organ, tissue, and eye donations which would come much later. I focused instead on my belief that he was alive in Heaven.

As I read the obituary in the newspaper the next day, August 6th, I stared in disbelief. This can't be!! He is too young! Maybe someone will tell me this is a bad dream, but no one ever did!

And yet, I momentarily forgot his wish, "If anything happens to me, I want to donate my organs so others will live…" Organ donation would be Tom's legacy, his request fulfilled, an honor bestowed as four lives were saved and others enhanced. I would never know how far-reaching this decision would be until I met Tom's heart recipient. Let me introduce you to Pete Radigan.

PART II

Pete's Story

4

Meeting Pete Radigan

In 1997, Edmund Peter Radigan III was not an upstate New Yorker, a motorcycle rider, or even a teenager. By most accounts, his life was relatively calm and easier to navigate than the young man who would become spiritually and physically intertwined with him.

Pete resided in of East Windsor, New Jersey, born in Staten Island, New York in 1965 as the oldest child, and only son, among the five children of Mickey and Ellen Radigan—two sales professionals who possessed large hearts, personalities, and gifts of gab worthy of a kissing trip to the Blarney Stone. His sisters' names were indicative of a large Irish-Catholic family—Kerry, Tracy, Jeanie, and Jennifer.

Mickey and Ellen met when he was a student-athlete at Wagner College on Staten Island during the early 1960s. Mickey played basketball for the Seahawks and was part of the 1963-64 team that upset #7 ranked NYU at the old Sutter Gymnasium.

By all accounts, Pete's early childhood was normal. The Radigan brood were all vested in sports, and each sister eventually earned a Division I athletic scholarship in basketball or field hockey. As a youngster, Pete involved himself in tackle football, wiffleball, and played along with any game taking place among his immediate relatives and nearly two dozen first cousins in the large Radigan backyard.

As Pete said, "We grew up in a super big Irish Catholic family." Every July 4th, the sports accompanied those who came to the house for the annual Independence Day party, which included basketball tournaments in the driveway, swimming in the family pool, and selected games on the grass.

Mickey kept the family in the game through his coaching involvement in the Police Athletic League (PAL), which continued until Pete's preteens.

Yet, as young Pete worked his way through grammar school, it became apparent he suffered from severe physical limitations. "Exercise never felt good," he admitted. In retrospect, the teenager managed to play tennis in high school, mainly because "it did not involve consistent running, but having form, which he excelled at.He could nail the ball and put a straight shot down the lines almost as hard as a pro player."

However, the physical limitations came into full view after high school. Pete followed in his father's footsteps and made the decision to attend Wagner. But unlike the flat landscape of central Jersey, Wagner perched itself atop Grymes Hill, the highest point on the eastern seaboard. Not only were the hills steep, but the paths to the campus were also long, with a half to three-quarter mile route to get up either side. Even a walk from his dorm, Harbor View Hall, to the Union building was a gradient uphill slope of roughly 35 degrees.

"I used to plan my day around making that trip," confessed Pete, possibly for the first time ever, and 30 years after college. "If I had to go to the library or to class, I would bring everything with me so I would not have to go back to my room and walk that hill again."

Socially, Pete's aversion to heavy physical activity was not a factor. As a first-semester freshman, he pledged the Tau Kappa Epsilon (TKE) fraternity. Pledge activities were grueling but usually centered on the candidate's ability to chug beer and memorize important facts about one's pledge classmates. "Trenton! Mahwah! Yorktown Heights! Utica! Sir!!" was part of an enduring chant among the pledge class as they rattled off the hometowns of their brothers-to-be.

But TKE was the party fraternity at Wagner, and where the brothers went, so did the beer. The chapter lounge, nestled at the right end of a nondescript concrete hallway underneath Cunard Hall, was dank, dark, and smelled like stale Budweiser but was always filled to near capacity whenever a keg arrived. The local bars down the back hill were Pop's, Corner Inn, and Brandy's, which also kept their businesses thriving during the school months as fraternity brothers and sorority sisters came to play shuffleboard and drink endless pitchers.

Pete drove a car on campus early in his collegiate career, but it was not to show independence or dare the Staten Island police to pull him over at 4:00 a.m. There was an unknown secret bottled inside the young frater.

"I was scared to death," said Pete. "Whenever we went down the back hill to a bar, I always drove." Thinking more about his answer, he continued, "I was afraid one night I would get stuck in Brandy's or Corner Inn without a ride back to school and have to walk up that hill. I physically could not walk up that hill and felt fearful I would be stuck somewhere in between during the middle of the night."

Being in the era before cell phones, the fear was real, just like the threat of becoming a crime victim as the bars were located on or near Richmond Road, Targee Street, and Vanderbilt Avenue, which bordered the Park Hill projects. The projects were later made famous through the songs and stories of the Wu-Tang Clan, but in the early 1980s, it was the Force MD's ("Tender Love"), who would make trips up the back hill from their collective home in the projects to the Wagner campus to dazzle students with their brand of a cappella.

While awaiting the implantation of a new heart in 1997, Pete started to reflect on his life. Here is how he described his developing years and the events that led to his life-changing operation.

Pete's Diary Prologue

"For as long as I can remember, I have always been part of a family that has loved and cherished every moment we have together. My mother, Ellen, and my father, Mickey, were insistent on good behavior but led by example for all of us. I was also blessed with four sisters, Kerry, Tracey, Jeanie, and Jennifer. You may have heard the colloquialism that says, "My family is everything." I can honestly say I live that every day. Since the events of the last four years of my life, my family is even more important than before.

I was born with tight joints, short hamstrings, and a heart murmur. These things happen, but I grew up living a normal and active childhood. I was never as athletic as my sisters who were all collegiate athletes in different sports. This did not bother me because I had more fun than you will ever know being involved in amateur athletics, bowling, and especially tennis.

I excelled in the sport of tennis. I could not get enough of it. It started with lessons, then playing with Mom and Dad, and grew into an obsession I loved.

My life was happy and healthy until things came to a screeching halt in April of 1987. You see, I went on an exchange program with my college, Wagner College, on Staten Island. Prior to leaving for Bregenz, Austria, in August of 1986, I passed a physical by a physician who pronounced me fit to travel and participate in the exchange program. However, when I returned the troubles began.

I returned from my exchange experience in January 1987, but approximately two months later I started getting sick. Over a two-month period, I contracted strep throat once and bronchitis several times. The last time I went to consult with Dr. Robert Aitken, he told me my heart sounded like a herd of horses and he was unsure why. This was disturbing to my doctor because he heard nothing out of the ordinary before I left for Europe. I was sent to Princeton Medical Center for an echocardiogram. Dr. Manuel T. Amendo, who is now my local cardiologist, evaluated my echocardiogram. He later told Dr. Aitken that my heart had increased in size, and I needed a cardiac catheterization to determine if there was any damage.

I decided to go to the Philadelphia Heart Institute to undergo a heart catheterization. The catheterization, which is not a difficult procedure, produced an infection at the site of the catheter in the artery in my right arm. The results of the heart catheterization came back inconclusive, with no answer for my heart's behavior or the unexplained thickness in the walls of my heart.

Dr. Aitken was disturbed by this and wrote to the head of the heart institute at the National Institute of Health to ask them to accept me into their program to determine the cause of the problem. Several months later, they notified me that I had been accepted into their program.

I was 21 years old at the time and I felt like I was invincible, so I did not feel concerned because I did not feel bad. The doctors kept indicating something was not right; but if you feel good, this does not create much of an impact on your life.

In April of 1987, I entered the National Institute of Health in Bethesda, Maryland, to be evaluated to determine the cause of the heart issues. It was decided when I graduated or finished college in June that I would undergo a heart biopsy to determine the heart issues. Because I felt good, I did not even feel the slightest bit concerned as stated previously.

In early August, the physician admitted me into Bethesda Naval Hospital at the National Institute of Health to undergo the heart biopsy. For the first time, I really observed the tension on my mother and father's faces. This observation was the first of what I now believe would be a life-long worry regarding how the course of my health would ultimately impact my family.

Finally, a diagnosis. The results were identified as a heart disease called Hypertrophic Cardiomyopathy (HCM). I did not know it then, but this was the disease that would change the course of my life forever."

5

Pete's Story - December 1995

"I remember saying to myself that early December morning, "Man, my feet have been really hurting off and on for the last several months. When I get back from this trip, I will check this out with my physician.""

Over the past several months, my doctor had sent me to a rheumatoid doctor to care for my feet as I often experienced gout. I always thought it was just a side effect of the low dose of diuretics I took for my heart disease. The doctors usually treated it, and within a few days, the pain associated with the swelling from gout went away. The only problem was that the frequency of the episodes had increased exponentially over the last several months.

The rheumatoid doctor became concerned, as well, and decided to send me for a muscle biopsy to check for a muscle/skin disease called Dermatomyositis. He had several reasons for assuming this disease may be present. The first was the red/purplish color which became more pronounced on my knees, elbows, and joints. The second reason was I experienced constant aching at the joints, which they thought was gout.

The muscle biopsy turned out to be negative, and the doctors diagnosed what I had as Asymptomatic Dermatomyositis. This means that although the muscle biopsy showed no signs of the disease, the skin clearly indicated it was present.

The rheumatoid doctor then began a course of treatment with a powerful medication called Prednisone. Even today, I wonder if this course of treatment for an asymptomatic disease helped to push forward an impending heart failure that would occur less than a month and a half later. You see, Prednisone retains salt, which retains fluid in the body. When your body goes into heart failure, your heart is not functioning properly, and you retain fluid.

The redness/purpleness in my joints had always been there. It always seemed to be worse in the winter with the dry air. During the summer months when I was outside in the sun, the redness/purpleness seemed to be virtually gone one day and there the next day. There seemed to be no rhyme or reason for why it was happening.

My conjecture is that my heart failure was the cause of the redness/purpleness due to a problem with circulation within my diseased heart. The redness/purpleness was not rough or in any way a rash. As a matter of fact, when you pressed that area on the skin, it would clear up and then return. It reacted the same way as when you squeeze your finger and it turns red and then when you touch it, the tip clears up before turning red again.

These were the preceding events leading up to the January that will live in infamy in my life as well as my family's.

January 1996

The month started out fantastically. I traveled quite a bit, and enjoyed being single. Where else can you do what you love to do for a living and travel around the country, as well? It was during the third week of the month when my problems began.

The third week in January of 1996 was a week that I will never forget for the rest of my life. I was traveling from Newark, New Jersey to

Orange County, California via a connecting flight out of Houston, Texas. I had my usual traveling stuff—my training bag, my computer, and as usual, carried these things through the airport. My gate was located in the lower-left sector of the airport, and my connection was in the upper right. When I departed the plane, I started walking towards my connecting flight. As I I walked past two gates in the airport, I could not catch my breath as I also started sweating. When this is happening, the mentality of a 30-year-old is, *How did I get so out of shape so quickly?*

I know it sounds bad, but although I was walking slowly and laboriously, I really felt like I was just getting the flu and would be fine if I could just get to California. This was going to be a long week if I became sick. My saving grace was I was in the final stages of cross-training another trainer and would not be on the platform for long stretches. Therefore, I concluded if I became sick, I could probably struggle through it. At this point in my career, I was an accomplished Instructional Designer and a trainer with strong facilitation skills that enabled me to teach what I had written. In this case, I had designed a behavior management training program for Ricoh's sales managers. Because I designed the training program, I also facilitated the Train-the-Trainer (T3). This is what brought me to California.

When I arrived at the hotel, I still felt awful. My problems did not end there. The faulty air conditioning unit in my room did not work, and I felt sick and hot at the same time. If you have ever had the flu, you know this is a nasty combination.

I started teaching the class the next day. When I arrived at my West Coast training center, I had to walk up one flight of stairs. This proved to be a 15-minute task as I had to stop three times to catch my breath. Again, I assumed it was the flu. I knew this was going to be a tough day.

As the day progressed, I taught certain modules. I literally taught for two hours then took a 15-minute break, went to the office, and slept for 20 minutes. The instructor from the West Coast then woke me up, and I taught for another two hours before breaking for lunch for an hour. During that time I slept, as well, and the instructor had to once again wake me up. This went on throughout the rest of the day and for the next four days. I did not know it then, but I had been having right heart failure the whole week. In addition to all of this, at the end of the four days, my feet excessively swelled, and I struggled to walk. My first thought was I was having another gout attack. Little did I know, but the swelling of my feet over the last several months was not gout but the beginning stages of heart failure.

I finished the class and, despite everything, received top ratings for the class. This became the rating joke of the year within my company. "Nobody should ever complain about ratings because Pete had heart failure and got top ratings" was the comment of the year. My last comment to my boss was that I planned to return home, stay out of work until I figured out the problem when I returned to New Jersey.

When I got home, I found the swelling in my feet had increased. I failed to urinate, and my feet doubled in size. Due to this, I could not wear regular shoes. I also struggled with swallowing for some reason, like I had a lump in my throat. It felt like I was trying to swallow a piece of steak but was unable to get it down my throat.

The only problem was I was not eating anything at all. I felt really scared. It felt like someone closing your throat forcefully but still being able to breathe; but when you tried to breathe, you gagged. My primary physician, Dr. Lynn Kossow, was concerned enough that she sent me to a breathing specialist for an examination. Additionally, she increased my diuretic to drain some of the fluid buildup. When I went to the breathing specialist, I could barely walk. They transported me in a wheelchair, and the specialist focused on my feet so he did not even evaluate my breathing problem other than to discuss it. He called Dr. Kossow who admitted me immediately into Princeton Medical Center. And then the problems really began.

At this point in time, no one really understood how bad it was. Frankly, I wasn't sure so I didn't make a big deal out of it. My mother and father were concerned but mainly because I was clearly sick and dating a woman who my mom didn't think would take proper care of me. My mother wanted me to stay at their home, instead of my home, to make sure I was alright.. I did not think it was anything to worry about so I declined her offer. When she took me to the doctor she saw firsthand how much pain I was really in.

When I was admitted into Princeton Medical Center, I had another echocardiogram. Dr. Amendo compared it with the previous echocardiogram I had nine years earlier, when I was originally diagnosed with heart disease. When the results came back, the thickness of the wall of my right heart had doubled in size. This, as I later learned, was the reason I had gone into heart failure. Dr. Amendo ordered a whole gamut of tests to determine my heart problems.

It was late on the third day in the hospital when Drs. Kossow and Amendo came into my room with the results of the tests and news that would change my life forever. As you recall, I come from a really big Irish family. Drs. Kossow and Amendo both stood about 5'4" and were surrounded by a family of 12-14 people averaging 5'10" and taller to hear the news of my condition. It was at this point I received the most sobering statement that anyone could tell me in my life.

The physicians told me I experienced right heart failure causing me to gain 30 pounds of water and experience shortness of breath, as my girlfriend and my family surrounded me. I said, "Okay, so what medication do I take to help or fix the condition?"

The doctors then told me, "You don't understand. We can give you medication to try to keep you alive, but without a heart transplant you will die."

There was a collective gasp by my family. Imagine your only son and brother being told he is dying when only a few months ago he was running around like normal? Thinking back, I can honestly say if there is one thing I could take away from this experience, it would be the impact this had on my family. I knew at that time that my death would have a crippling effect on my family, at least in the short term.

At the time, I had been dating a woman for about eight months; and when she met me, I felt vibrant and energetic. Now, eight months later, she was dating a man who needed a heart transplant. I did not know if she planned to see this ordeal through or even if she would want to. Due to my impending struggles, I did not want to think about it. She would either hang in there and recognize when I received the transplant, I would be healthy again or she may not. I knew only time would tell.

When you are 30 years old, this is not something readily acceptable to you. Your mentality is that this does not happen to you, this happens to other people. This happens to people much older than you who do not take care of themselves. The reality of the situation, as I have come to realize over the last four years, is this can happen to infants, teenagers, young and older adults, as well. There is no rhyme or reason for why it happens.

Once I had accepted the fact that I indeed needed a heart transplant to survive, I said to the doctors, "Alright, if this is what I need to do to live, let's do it! Let's get it over with so I can go on with my life!"

Their response was very measured. I could tell how uncomfortable they were as they said, "You can't just take a heart off a shelf. You have to be evaluated to see if you are a candidate for a heart transplant, and only then will you be placed on a waiting list."

I was amazed at this response and said, "Did you just tell me if I don't receive a transplant I will die?"

They said, "Yes, but there are thousands of others like you waiting. You need to go through the process. They will give you medications to stabilize you during the wait." Imagine being told you are dying and in the same breath being told to wait. Imagine if I were not talking about my situation but that of a loved one. You can understand how frustrated and helpless I felt at that moment.

Let me explain about the "Waiting List" with regards to organ donation. The "Waiting List" is a nationwide list governed by The United Network of Organ Sharing (UNOS). There are many factors determining who will obtain an organ and when. Those factors include the severity of your health, blood type, size, and antibodies (which are proteins used by the immune system to identify and neutralize foreign objects such as bacteria and viruses which could cause rejection of the organ). Despite what many people think, money does not play a factor. Many people believe Mickey Mantle received an organ quickly because he was a celebrity. This is unequivocally not true. He referred himself to multiple transplant centers and could travel to these locations within an hour if they contacted him for a transplant. Even though he had the financial means to be active at the transplant centers, he did not pay to be moved up on the list.

Another example is Frank Torre, the brother of Joe Torre, the former New York Yankees manager. Many people thought he received his heart quickly because he was the brother of Joe Torre and an ex-professional athlete. When Frank's story came out in the newspaper, most people did not know he was dying and waited for over three months for his transplant in the hospital.

The next day my doctors released me in a wheelchair from Princeton Medical Center with a phone number to Dr. Donna Mancini, the transplant specialist at Columbia Presbyterian Medical Center, to make an appointment to be evaluated. Dr. Mancini, along with Dr. Robert Micheler, would ultimately be the ones who saved my life and continue to save my life to this day.

Imagine being a mother and seeing your only son go from healthy to barely being able to walk and not knowing why.

February 1996

My first trip up to Columbia Presbyterian Medical Center was a painful one. I gained over 30 pounds of water weight that literally seeped through my skin around my ankles. At this point, I could barely walk. My parents' concerned looks became obvious even though they tried to maintain a strong front and appearance. My dad went into the hospital and found a wheelchair to transport me to the 14th-floor transplant clinic to Dr. Mancini's office.

Imagine a frightened 30-year-old, who for the first time was terrified of the unknown. As a child growing up, I felt invincible. Nothing bad can happen to you because it always happens to someone else. As scared as I was, I held my feelings inside because I knew my family felt equally, if not more, concerned and fearful they could lose me. Waiting, which is a word you will read constantly throughout these events, became the worst part and is the worst part for most transplant recipients.

In retrospect, waiting for Dr. Mancini to tell me exactly what was wrong with me was the worst feeling, especially when she confirmed that Drs. Amendo's and Kossow's diagnosis of heart failure was true. Dr. Mancini did not say I would be placed on the waiting list, but I would be admitted and evaluated to see if I would be a candidate for a heart transplant. She seemed confident I would be placed on the list but did not commit herself to yes or no. This really bothered me because I knew that if I did not receive a heart transplant, I would surely die.

I was not ready to accept this as the truth. Once again, I had to keep my fear inside. I never thought for a minute I would not survive. However, I did not feel ready to handle the impact my death would have on my family. The more I waited without knowing my prognosis, the worse my mindset became.

By the time I had reached Dr. Mancini's office, my slippers were saturated with water to the point that I could have rung them out like wet rags. I was in obvious pain and in obvious jeopardy.

Dr. Mancini came in, and her first comment was hysterical. Dr. Mancini has a dry serious tone, but it was her comment that took the house down! I had my mom, dad, and Mrs. McFadden, my mom's close friend, with me in the room. Dr. Mancini's first question was, "Pete, is this your mother, father, and grandmother?" My mom put her head down, but you could see her body quivering in hysterical laughter as she tried to keep it under control.

All I said was, "No, this is my mom's friend." This only caused my mom to laugh harder and Mrs. Fadden's anger to grow. By the time

Dr. Mancini left the room, my mom could barely breathe. When Dr. Mancini finally left, Mrs. McFadden mumbled, "I am going to @#%& kill her!" This is the one early story that lives on with laughter 20+ years later.

Dr. Mancini examined me and immediately decided that I needed to be evaluated for a cardiac heart transplant. She was concerned about the diagnosis of Asymptomatic Dermatomyositis. This is a disease of the skin and the muscles. As I previously mentioned, I had a muscle biopsy in December that came back negative for Dermatomyositis. My symptoms included red and purplish coloring on my knees and elbows. Yet, all tests came back negative. If this disease was present and active, the doctors and Columbia may not be willing to place me on the transplant list to give me a lifesaving heart transplant. This was a scary thought because my parents and I knew that without the heart transplant I would die. It took several weeks for them to rule this out. Once again, the waiting came into play and added stress for both my family and me.

Dr. Mancini asked, "Do you want to go home or wait to see if I can admit you into the hospital for evaluation?" Since I could not walk, I immediately decided this was a "no brainer." I would wait to see if she could admit me to the hospital which occurred on February 7, 1996. This began my transplant saga at Columbia Presbyterian Medical Center. This first stay at Columbia ended up being just over four weeks in the hospital. The Columbia cardiac floor was the sixth floor in the Milstein Hospital Building in New York.

At this stage of my life, I had never been in the hospital for an extended stay. I never had the opportunity or recognized the value of the medical and nursing staff. These people really make the hospital click. My stay would have been a living hell if these caregivers did not have such patience and love towards their patients no matter what their race, creed, religious background, or otherwise. There were no barriers, just unconditional caring. My ability to wait, as well as the ability of others to survive the stress of the wait, can be attributed to the nursing staff of the sixth and seventh floor at Columbia Presbyterian Medical Center. Columbia's nursing staff was outstanding! Their commitment to quality is evident in the fact that I am alive and strong today.

The first order of business for the doctors at Columbia was to drain my body of the 30 pounds of excess fluids that had built up due to the heart failure. No cardiac transplant could take place until this was corrected. I needed to be on an intravenous medication (IV) called Dobutamine to stabilize my heart failure and be placed on the transplant list for Status 1. Status 1 is when a person awaiting a transplant is among the sickest in the nation and at the top of the UNOS (United Network for Organ Sharing) waiting list for their organ transplant or organ transplants. Remember, UNOS is the keeper of the national list for all those waiting for transplants irrespective of the transplantable organ. Dobutamine is prescribed to patients experiencing heart failure to increase the efficiency of the heart and reduce the symptoms of heart failure. As bad as I felt when I came in, this Dobutamine acts like a miracle drug for heart failure patients. Remember, I struggled to breathe and retained fluid at the time of admission. The doctor prescribed Lasix, a powerful diuretic, to work with the Dobutamine and drain the excess fluid. I took Lasix 200 mg twice daily. Since this is a high dose, I took 13 tablets of K-Dur 20 Meq. (milequivalents) to compensate for the loss in potassium caused by the high dose of Lasix. After about 24 hours on the Dobutamine and Lasix, I had the greatest relief ever. I started urinating a lot. Imagine being happy about going to the bathroom? I felt ecstatic!

Because I had gained over 30 pounds in water weight from the heart failure, it took the better part of three weeks to remove the excess fluid. The worst part of the fluid draining came right near the end of the process. When most of the fluid had been removed, my skin began to itch incredibly. This was a direct result of the expansion of my skin around my ankles and a quick and drastic reduction of weight in a short period of time. This was unlike any bad itching I have ever experienced in my life. You may be able to relate if you have ever experienced a slight sunburn when your skin lifts and causes itching. Well, that lasts for a short period of time and goes away. Try to magnify that feeling 15 times without relief for a day and a half. The itching was so bad that I lacerated my skin around both ankles to the point the medical staff wrapped it to control the bleeding.

To make matters worse, now that the swelling had subsided, I thought I should be able to walk. You would think this would be logical. No more swelling—stand up and walk, right? Wrong! The effects of the itching on my ankles and the need to remove more fluid for about three more days contributed to the reason that I could not stand up. When I attempted to, more excess fluid drained to my ankles and sent the most incredible burning sensation to my ankles which produced excruciating pain. The lacerations around my ankles felt like the ground separating during an earthquake for weeks. I forgot about walking for about another week.

Finally, after 3½ weeks from the first day I entered Columbia, the 30 pounds of fluid was removed and I returned to some semblance of feeling normal.

My feet were still sore from the lacerations, but I finally walked again for the first time in almost a month. You tend to take for granted the gifts you have been given, such as walking, breathing, sweating, etc.until you no longer have that 100% of the time. When I became capable of walking, I felt even more grateful for the gifts God gave me. I knew there was a long road ahead of me. I began to understand the importance of God, family, close friends of the family, close business friends, colleagues, etc., and the impact they would have on my life and ultimately my ordeal and recovery. This mindset, in hindsight, was a great attitude to have. It never entered my mind that I would not survive.

Now there were other issues going on here besides the fluid around my ankles. One of which was Dermatomyositis. Dad had picked up my muscle biopsy results from Princeton Medical Center because most doctors chose to individually evaluate and review results for themselves. Columbia's doctors were no different. They were some of the best doctors in the world, and I would come to realize they would leave no stone unturned. The dermatology doctors evaluating the muscle biopsies agreed with the Asymptomatic Dermatomyositis. This was great news. If the doctors thought it was symptomatic and would eventually attack the muscles, they would not have allowed me to be placed on the transplant list. This was the second major hurdle they resolved so I could ultimately receive my life-saving heart transplant.

During the third week in the hospital, I hit a major roadblock. I had a fever of over 100 degrees. This was considered a slight fever, but due to my normal low blood pressure, the doctors transferred me to the Coronary Intensive Care Unit (CICU). When a person is in heart failure, the pressures within the heart can elevate to dangerous levels. My pressures were extremely high. Since being admitted into the hospital, I endured four cardiac catheterizations. The doctors could not bring down my pressures to an acceptable level to place me on the transplant waiting list.

I was not willing to consider the fact that I might not be able to receive a heart transplant. My parents, family, and doctors kept this very real possibility from me. During the second week, a member of the transplant team, Dr. Howard Levin, visited. Dr. Levin made this first part of my ordeal tolerable. He always came in with jokes, sarcasm, and kept the mood light. He could always find good news in what appeared to be a negative or hopeless situation.

During this hospital stay, my family was a brick wall of support. They left no stone unturned when it came to one of them being there for me. I cannot imagine what it would have been like not having the type of family support that I had throughout this ordeal. But it was not easy for everybody in my life. My girlfriend began to struggle with handling things. I saw her occasionally but was struggling with dealing with my situation. Even though she claimed to love me, I began to realize she may not be the one for me. I had to honestly tell myself I did not know how I would react if I was in a similar situation.

While I was in CICU, I did my best to present a strong front to my parents and most of my family. I did not want them to think I even entertained the possibility that I would not survive, even though I knew this could be a very real possibility. Throughout my life, I have always been close to my sisters. However, I felt closest to my sister,

Tracey. We could talk about everything. That had its good points and its bad points. Unfortunately for her, one of the bad points would occur during my transplant ordeal. Remember, I did not want my family to know that I ever thought there was any possibility I would not survive? With that in mind, I kept my feelings and thoughts inside. My fears were mounting by the day. I felt angry this could happen to me along with other intense feelings associated with my new reality. My family staggered in at different times to visit me. The advantage of having a large family during my hospital stay is they could plan their visits so someone was present with me most of the time. I cannot remember more than a day when someone from my family did not visit. About every four days, Tracey and my brother-in-law Pat would visit. When Tracey came, I would ask her to talk to me alone; and without fail, I broke down hysterically crying. I always took pride in the control of my life, and here I was crying like a baby. Tracey was great. Despite how upset and emotional she became from seeing me so upset, she listened and gave me the best advice she could. I do not know if she realizes how much this support meant to me at that time. Recounting this story still triggers strong emotions for me. Imagine being Tracey and knowing she visited her brother who was dying and having him break down in tears every time she came. Yet she remained strong and continued to visit me, nonetheless. For that and many other things, I love her very much.

One of the hardest conversations I had during this whole ordeal was with my parents during my stay in CICU. I discussed with them what to do if I did not survive. We were all upset as you can imagine during this conversation. My father said to me, "We'll talk about this once and then we will not talk about it again."

I said, "Okay. If for some reason I do not survive this situation, this is what I want you to do. I want you to split everything I own and try to pay off what you can of your mortgage along with my sisters' mortgages. Do what you need to mourn, but then I want you to have a massive party and celebrate my life as it was, not as it is in death. Okay?" At this point, all three of us were an emotional mess. Many people are envious of our family. All my life, I can be out with my parents or any one of my sisters and have as good a time as with the best of my friends. My family is not only my family, but they are my best friends.

You never know how many people you have touched in your life until a tragic event like this occurs. During my stay in the hospital, I received hundreds of letters from people I trained on my job and others whose lives I touched during my young life. These people included immediate family, close friends, distant friends, work associates, work acquaintances, etc. It felt comforting to know I could count on them for support. This, even today, helps me to understand how important a support system can be during a traumatic event in your life.

At one point in CICU when I had a fever and was finally told about the possibility that I would not be put on the list, I asked for my parents to bring Father Pat Castles to the hospital to see me. Now, Father Pat was not a people person; but I wanted him to come, hear my confession, and give me a blessing for the sick. I remember my mom, who is as sarcastic as me, asking Father Pat if he could come to visit me. He replied that he could not come and asked if there was a minister in the hospital? She said to him, "My son is dying and I am coming to get you now. Be ready!" And he was ready.

Father Pat arrived and we talked. I felt upset as I gave him my confession, and he asked me if I wanted rites for the sick. My immediate statement to him was, "No, I'm not dying!"

He said, "Many people think that, but it is just a blessing for people who are sick."

I then replied, "Thank you and please." With that, Fr. Pat gave me the blessing for the sick.

You know, I have always been religious, but nothing would have prepared me for the events of the next week.

Remember, at this time they were thinking I may not be able to receive a transplant if the pressure around my heart did not return to an acceptable level. Even if they placed me on the transplant list, I would probably have to wait in the hospital until I received the heart. I thought I may not be able to attend my sister Jeanie's impending wedding which was coming up two months later in April. Within ten days after Father Pat gave me the blessing for the sick, I stabilized. My blood pressure normalized. With the use of a medication called Nipride, it brought down the pressures within my heart. Finally, I was placed on the waiting list for a heart transplant after almost four weeks of evaluation. I had stabilized so well that the doctors were able to wean me off the Dobutamine while all my pressures and everything else stayed in a safe range.

Miraculously, on March 6, 1996, I was released from the hospital taking 35 pills a day to keep me stable. I was placed on the United Network for Organ Sharing (UNOS) transplant waiting list, Status 2. Status 1 means you are the highest priority and among the most sick in the nation waiting for your respective organ for transplant. Status 2 meant I was accruing time on the UNOS waiting list that would be counted in the event I went to Status 1.

Please understand the fact that I was discharged with a price tag. My prescriptions included massive doses of diuretics and potassium to keep the heart failure and heart pressures at bay. I took about 35 different pills a day to keep myself stable. This I did for the better part of fifteen months while I was Status 2.

I attended my sister, Jeanie's wedding, which became the best part of my hospital discharge. I not only attended her wedding but said the nuptial prayer, as well.

March - April 1996

The expression, "Home Sweet Home" was so apropos for my first trip home pre-transplant. That was the expression that came to mind when I walked through my parents' front door. My feet were still wrapped and healing from the lacerations, but things were starting to get back to some semblance of normalcy.

When I left the hospital, I asked Dr. Mancini if I could return to work while I waited for the heart. Imagine, I was about to go through the most dangerous surgery in my entire life and I wanted to go back to work. She said, "Let's wait and see how you do, and we will talk about it next month."

I still felt nervous when I arrived at my parents' house. Even though I could walk, I did not feel normal yet. I became a "couch potato" for the first couple of weeks in March. My medications stabilized me and helped me to think the impending transplant may be a possibility. I felt good. Once my ankles completely healed, I would feel as if things were almost back to normal.

My girlfriend worked nearby, and she would come from my house to my parents' house at night. Remember, she knew me as energetic. But by the time the night rolled around, I felt exhausted. Even though I may not have done much during the day, I still became tired. I felt frustrated and emotional as I adjusted to this change. We began to argue more and more. She wanted the energetic Pete she had met nearly nine months ago. I wanted to be that person, but until I received the transplant, that would not happen. I knew I could be on the medication for a while and may not receive the transplant right away. She stated that she wanted me to receive the transplant right away so I could return to my previous self and engage in activities with her. My family felt downright angry with her for making that statement. They felt having me somewhat healthy but on a lot of medication was better than going through a major surgery in which I might not survive. After I heard about this conversation, I admitted I felt angry as well, agreeing with my family. She was being selfish, and I could not accept that. I began to think this relationship may not work out as I thought of ways to end it painlessly.

Towards the end of March, Jeanie had been in the final stages of planning for her wedding to Joe Felipe, who is now my brother-in-law. My feet had pretty much healed, and I was moving around easier. I cannot tell you how good it felt. Additionally, I had moved back to my own house.

I lived in a development about five minutes from my parents. I felt truly blessed to have the neighbors that I did. Hans and Michele Schumacher and Pedro and Fiona Rodriguez were like an extended family to me. While I was in the hospital, Hans and Michele, who loved yard work and fixing things around the house, helped me immensely. They were available for anything I ever needed. Three or four times a week we either ate at their house or at mine. Over the years, we have become the greatest of friends. Pedro and Fiona were just as willing to help, except they did not do yard work. They had one son, Thomas, who was a great kid. When I first returned to my home, they were always there to provide support.

As April 1996 rolled around, I felt nearly healthy again. All things considered, it almost makes me chuckle to say I was nearly healthy. I took tons of medication, but my ankles healed. I walked with relatively no problems. I thought about returning to work. Yet, in my mind, I did not want to jeopardize my health. I already decided my life was in Dr. Mancini's hands. Whatever she said or decided would be the law for me.

I met with Dr. Mancini for my clinic visit during the first week in April and she asked me how I was feeling. I told her I urinated a lot (which was a good thing in my case) and felt great. She said I was doing well and to continue as is.

I asked her at this point again if there was a possibility that I could return to work because I was starting to go crazy back at my house doing nothing. Dr. Mancini kind of laughed and said, "Do you really want to go back?"

I replied, "Doc, I don't want to put my health in jeopardy; and if you say that I will put myself in jeopardy by going back to work, then I will not. However, if I can, it will mentally help me quite a bit."

She said, "Would you consider going back part-time?"

I told her that I did not think my company would allow that. Then I thought of a possible compromise. "What if my company were to allow me to develop curriculum and work 20 hours a week at the office and 20 hours a week at home on my computer. Would that be acceptable health-wise for you?"

Dr. Mancini smiled and said, "We'll try it and see how you feel."

I was ecstatic. I still took a lot of medication, but I planned to return to work and would continue while I waited for my pending transplant. My company agreed and made the necessary accommodations for me. I never realized that I had a talent for writing until this happened to me. Developing curriculum gave me the chance to enhance this ability and to recognize other talents I possessed. This was just another way of expanding my professional boundaries and capabilities.

My life started coming together again. I planned to return to work on May 6, 1996, and I felt happy as a clam. Jeanie and Joe's wedding weekend came on April 28th. I cannot tell you how happy I felt to be present at their wedding. I come from a really big Irish family and about 160 of the guests were immediate family and close friends on our side of the family. News of my health situation had spread like wildfire. Between my family and me, we received hundreds of calls concerning my health and wellbeing. At the wedding, everyone was overjoyed that I was able to attend. I remember when I said the prayer, I made a joke about transplants to lighten everyone's fear about the process of going through a heart transplant.

I also found many people could not fathom the struggle I faced. I knew I had to lighten the tension everyone felt but could not express to my family and myself. My plan of making light of the situation helped everyone cope better. I find that ironic even today. Ironic in that I was the one who was going to go through the major surgery, yet my family feared for me almost as much as I did. Personally, it never entered my mind when I left the hospital in February that I would not survive the surgery. Everyone else's fear was something I had to help them deal with. I kind of felt it was my responsibility to ease my family's fear about what I was about to endure. Afterward, everyone would tell me that my attitude was inspirational. I can honestly say I am just a realist and care as much about my family as my life itself.

Jeanie and Joe's wedding was fantastic. We all had a blast and I danced and laughed and really had a good time with our whole family. After eight to ten hours of wedding festivities, although I felt good, I knew I was still in heart failure. I was exhausted and yet I was the happiest I had been in four months.

My girlfriend and I had finally had it out. She was continuing to have problems dealing with my health, and I could not handle her insecurity. Yet I felt bad about putting her in that position. One day while arguing on the phone, she said, "Do you want to continue going out?" That was my out.

I said, "You know what, I do not think we should continue to go out." That was it. Our nearly year-long relationship was over. Honestly, I never looked back. It was something I believe I should have done several months earlier but for some reason could not.

In less than a week I planned to return to work, and I could not wait.

May 1996

You know, it seems like every day that you are working, you think about your next vacation or day off. This is a part of everyday working life. After the events of the first four months of this year and having not worked in the same timeframe, I was eager to get back to work. Most people would think I was nuts. I received comments like, "Why don't you just enjoy yourself, rest, relax, etc.?" I can honestly say I am one of the few people that really loves what I do for a living. I love training and I love writing, as well.

On May 6th, after more than four months of being out of work, I returned to a workweek of 20 hours in the office and 20 hours at home. This was a great arrangement. I worked on revisions of two sales training curriculums for my company at home. Where necessary, I would intermittently fill in for some instructors, understanding that I could not spend eight hours on the platform, facilitating.

What I did not realize was the toll my working would have on me mentally. Although I enjoyed what I was doing and was working a reasonable schedule, I was still in heart failure. My mind told me I was fine and to continue doing the things that I did before my heart failure. The problem was my mind was writing checks my body could not cash. You see, when I worked for eight hours and finished, I felt exhausted and really could not physically do anything else for the rest of the day.

I remember going to my parents' house and telling them I felt exhausted and did not know why, but I had to go to sleep. This went on for the better part of the end of May and continued. I became emotional, frequently not knowing why. I remember my mom having an argument with my younger sister and feeling like I was being dragged into the middle of it. I got into my car and started crying. Remember, I am a 31-year-old man, and I am in my car crying for no apparent reason. This was not the first time this happened. I felt like I was starting to lose my mind. I had always taken great pride in having complete control of my life, career, and other parts of my life; now, I was breaking down for no plausible reason.

I remember questioning myself. Am I losing it? Do I need to get some help? My answers were almost a show of denial. No, I was not losing it! No, I do not need to get some help! But the question still haunted me, *Why were these things happening?* Why did they seem to be happening with more frequency? How could I find out without losing control of the life that I cherished so much? How would I find out without letting the world know that I was losing it? Or was I losing it at all?

I needed to talk about it to someone, so I called my sister, Tracey, and asked her to meet me for breakfast. She agreed and we met at a restaurant where I sat there and tried to explain how I felt.. Like the events of the last several weeks, I broke down and cried and struggled explaining why. I must say Tracey had become a pro at seeing me losing it, so this was becoming old hat.

We talked about why I felt I was losing it and why my emotions felt out of whack. She kept telling me I was going to have a heart transplant and anyone going through this would not be holding up half as well as I was. That did not help me, though. I felt like I was not holding it together when in the past I had no problem controlling my emotions and keeping them in check. I told her, "I am out of the hospital, I am working. Yes, I am more tired, but why am I reacting this way and crying for no apparent reason? This is not normal." She reiterated it was a normal reaction to everything I was going through and should be expected.

I told her that I was embarrassed to mention what I planned to tell her. I knew I did not need to say this to her, but I made her keep my plan confidential from family and friends. I told her I was considering consulting with a psychologist. She thought it was a good idea, and I should not be the slightest bit embarrassed about counseling. As a matter of fact, under the circumstances, she felt amazed I had not sought help prior to this time. She did say she thought everyone would be supportive of my plan since everyone loves me very much. At that time, I knew she was right. I almost felt guilty about not recognizing that others would support me.

So began the last summer before my transplant, while seeing a psychologist at the same time. What an interesting summer it was going to be.

Summer 1996

The summer of 1996 was the summer of the question, "Am I really losing my mind or not?" After my conversation with Tracey late in May, I decided to speak with a psychologist in my hometown of Hightstown, New Jersey. I felt really scared to consult with him. You might say, due to the events I had been through, how could this scare me any worse than the previous events that had taken place. I take great pride in being in control of things that happen in my life. I am not unrealistic. I do not think I can control everything. However, I have a great deal of self-confidence in myself and my abilities.

Back in April and May when my emotions started to get out of whack, I started doubting my ability to maintain control of my life. I was not sure why it was happening. This created a new stage of fear in my life.

When I decided to see the psychologist, I thought I was beginning down a road from which I may never find my way back. I had all kinds of questions prior to going into his office. Will I have to see this doctor forever? If I allowed him to get inside my head, would I be afraid of what he might tell me is wrong with me psychologically? If he does tell me what is wrong, should I or will I believe him? How difficult will it be to correct what is wrong with me? These were just some of the questions that were racing through my head at the time.

I had no idea just how far off-base I was about the psychologist's ability to help me. From the moment I went into his office, it was like a one-way rap session. He asked some open-ended questions about my life, and I just spouted, talking throughout the entire session. After two sessions, the doctor redefined stress for me. I am one of few people who can honestly say I love what I do. I love to train people. I love to present and speak publicly. I love to sell. These skills cause me to look forward to each day I work. The doctor asked me if I felt stressed at work or with my family. My answer was easy because I always felt that stress came from not feeling well, with events in work, or at life in general.

How wrong I was! After two weeks, the psychologist showed me stress did not just include my unhappiness with events at work or within my family life. Stress could also be the number of demands I place on myself both professionally and personally.

During my visits with the psychologist, subsequent to the stress conversations, he introduced me to stress tapes, or relaxation tapes. I always thought these relaxation tapes did not really work and people that used them were a bit crazy. The psychologist picked up my feelings through my hesitation and told me not to just take his word for it, but to try it and then decide.

What a pleasant surprise. Listening to this tape literally made me fall asleep and feel totally relaxed. I found it very ironic that I was introduced to hypnotherapy at Columbia Presbyterian when I was admitted for my final wait in the hospital. Hypnotherapy was similar in nature to the principles of the relaxation tapes. I found these then and even today to be a substantial benefit to me times when I feel things are crazy in my life.

I attended several sessions with the psychologist for the better part of a month during which he listened to me about everything in my life. I described my feelings regarding the upcoming transplant, my family, and my job.

I remember talking to the psychologist about my feelings regarding the fact that I had been bypassed twice for a management position at my company due to my health situation. This was very frustrating to me because I believed my credentials qualified me for this promotion. At one point, the hiring manager admitted one reason they did not offer the position was due to my declining health, although he could not officially cite this as a factor. But during the time I waited for my transplant, they bypassed me twice for the management position for the same reason—my health. Legally, when someone has a disability, that person cannot be treated differently; but nobody can tell me this is not the case. As fair and as well-intentioned people might be, the reality is "personal is personal" and "business is business." In my position, I was the most experienced with the best background, and yet twice during my disability I was overlooked for a management position for which I felt qualified. I think this was one of the most difficult things professionally I had to deal with while waiting for my transplant.

I don't blame them because you really need to take a lot of things, beyond just skillset, into consideration. When your mind is idle and you have no business frame of reference, it's hard and you create your own version of business stories. That being said, I was still upset at being overlooked but none more than when I returned back to work full time and was bypassed anyway even though I was more qualified.

Some of the most emotional times I spent talking with the psychologist were our conversations regarding my feelings surrounding my family. I described my intense feelings about the impact my potential death would have on my family as I relayed the extreme difficulty of my initial heart failure in February 1996. At multiple times during my recollection, I broke down and cried.

The discussions with the psychologist surrounding my upcoming transplant ended up being the final piece of my psychological puzzle. It was during these conversations that I realized the way I felt health-wise at that point was only temporary, and there was truly light at the end of the tunnel. It was this realization that helped me to understand that I really was not going crazy, but I just had to remember in my own mind that my health would improve upon completion of my transplant surgery.

Once I came to that realization, I ended therapy. I asked the psychologist at the end of this great epiphany when my next appointment would take place, and he said, "You are done."

I remember saying to him, "What do you mean, I'm done?" His response was simple. My fear was that my situation would always be this way. Until I came to the realization on my own that I had this fear, it would never be resolved. If the doctor had provided the answer instead, I may not have bought off on the realization. There is an adage that goes, "If you say it, it is a half-truth. If I say it, it is a whole truth." This saying really applies in my situation. Because I came up with the answer to my problem by myself, I realized I was not crazy but just going through a temporary process that in the end would bring normalcy back to my life.

Personally, with all the medications I was on, there were times I would almost forget I was in heart failure and on the waiting list for a transplant. I clearly remember one of the few times Dr. Mancini had gotten angry at me on the telephone. I was hanging around the pool with my sister Tracey and her husband Pat while he was waiting for my brother-in-law Scott to come over and play tennis. It was a beautiful and somewhat cool day, so I decided to warm Pat up until Scott got there on the tennis court. I felt great. Remember, the medications I was on were keeping my legs from swelling and retaining fluid, but I was on maximum doses of diuretics to keep me stable. I ended up not only warming him up but playing almost a full set of tennis before Scott arrived and I stopped.

Later that night when I got home, my ankles and feet swelled up. I thought I was having a recurrence of severe heart failure again, and I felt nervous and afraid. I called the transplant line at the hospital and talked with Dr. Mancini. I will never forget this incident. I informed Dr. Mancini my ankles swelled, but I had no fever. Then I said to her, "Would the fact I warmed up my brother-in-law on the tennis court have sent me into heart failure?"

She went the most ballistic I ever heard her. I clearly remember her comments even to this day. She said, "Did you forget you are in heart failure and although you feel good your medications prevent you from heart failure? If you do physical activity that increases your heart rate continually, your body and your heart are not strong enough to keep up. Unless you want to be admitted, I would strongly suggest you discontinue tennis until after the transplant." So ended my recreational career until after I received my transplant.

My company had been very good to me during this troubled time. They could have just dumped me or forced me to come to work every day or go out on disability and then terminate me in six months, but they chose not to do so. Although my colleagues, on the surface, said I would return to work, I could sense a change in their demeanor that questioned their sincerity. It was simply that my colleagues believed they may never see me again after the surgery. I was determined to prove them wrong!

The funny thing is, you cannot really blame anyone for the way they feel. My mother makes one of the truest statements I have ever heard, "Your feelings are not right or wrong, but they are your feelings, and you can't change the way you feel." When you think about it in the context of my work situation, you cannot really be that upset. I do not know if I would have reacted differently. Knowing how well I functioned, I definitely would act differently toward a person experiencing what I went through. The problem is you really cannot relate unless you personally have experienced it. This is the main reason why organ and tissue donation education is so important from a donor-recipient perspective.

I decided at that point that my professional career would have to be placed on the status quo until I recovered from the impending transplant. So went the summer of 1996.

Summer Turns to Fall, 1996

The fall brought new anxieties. Now, the reality of the upcoming transplant was beginning to set in. Starting in early summer, I asked Dr. Mancini where I was number-wise on the transplant list every time I visited. The reality of receiving a transplant is that waiting is the worst part of the whole experience. In June, Dr. Mancini told me that I was #16. In August, I was up to #9. In November, I was bumped down to #11.

This up and down movement was beginning to drive me crazy. I remember asking Dr. Mancini, "How is it that I can actually go down on the UNOS (United Network for Organ Sharing) waiting list instead of up or higher on the list?"

Her response was almost expected. "Hearts, as well as all organs, go to the sickest people first. You are Status 2. This means that you are sick, but the only way that you can consistently go up on the list is to be admitted into the hospital to be elevated to Status 1 which is considered the sickest people on the UNOS waiting list."

What a sinking feeling you have when you feel good (due to high doses of medication). Imagine being told that the only way to really get the organ you so desperately need is to spend immeasurable months inside the hospital awaiting the heart that could ultimately save your life.

Food was really starting to get on my nerves. You see, with heart failure, a low-sodium diet is imperative. Sodium, or salt, retains fluid, which counteracts the diuretics that are keeping your heart failure under control. A low-sodium diet for me meant no more than 1,000 milligrams of sodium per day. You might believe that this is not a big deal and that I should be able to handle it. I thought the same thing when I was told to change my diet. The problem is that there is so much sodium in everything we normally eat, a lack of salt would eliminate the taste in my diet. Salt is the one thing that adds taste to a lot of our food. So, what does this mean?

Imagine spending weeks trying to come up with a way that you could have pizza without making it high in sodium. I ended up using low-salt sauce, low-moisture, low-salt mozzarella, and spices on English Muffins. No more pizza from a restaurant until after the transplant, and even then, only very infrequently because of the fat restrictions.

There is salt in everything. Soup is high in salt. Rice dishes with any kind of flavoring are high in salt. Ham is high in salt. In supermarkets, it would take the better part of an hour just trying to count amounts of sodium in different meals to keep me near or below the 1,000 milligrams of sodium. The only good part of this is the weight loss that naturally comes with watching your diet and limiting your salt intake.

The Christmas of 1996 was a happy one for numerous reasons. For me, personally, I knew realistically that if things didn't work out I might not be here for the next Christmas. I knew this Christmas had to be one everyone remembered very well. I tried my best to keep my spirits up, but every time I thought about not being around or about dying, it literally would start driving me insane. Every time someone would toast to the fact that I was there and to my impending successful transplant and subsequent good health, it would nearly bring everyone to tears.

When I think back on it, I laugh. It was a time when everyone there put on a happy face while everyone thought the same thing. No one wanted to admit anything negative could or would happen, yet everyone knew the reality of my situation. The unsaid question in everyone's mind was, "Do you think Pete will be here next Christmas?" The answer everyone expressed verbally anytime the subject came up was, "Of course, he will. Look at all the successes. He is young, strong, etc." Imagine being in heart failure and having people say and think you are strong. It is the ultimate oxymoron.

Rolling Into 1997

I was starting to go a little bit bonkers at the beginning of January. I was still working at my company—twenty hours in the office and twenty hours outside the office. At the end of the day, I was still exhausted and really had no social life, but I still felt good. But once again, I would be reminded that God really does work in mysterious ways. This happened when Aroldo Rodriguez came into my life.

Just after the Christmas holiday, my aunt told me about a newspaper story regarding a local man who was in dire need of a heart transplant and was soon to be without medical insurance. It's funny how when things seem at their lowest point, God somehow finds a way to give you a renewed spirit and focus if you just give him the chance. He showed me the way by allowing me to reach out to offer support to Aroldo—words and thoughts from a person who was going through the same feelings and doubts at the same time, albeit for different reasons.

I first called Aroldo in mid-January 1997. We spoke briefly but agreed to talk again. Weeks later, after talking for some time, we agreed to meet. He lived three minutes from my house in the same town, and yet we were about to go through the same thing. Aroldo was in his late forties and a native of Colombia. He was an ex-Colombian League baseball player. Here we were—two people, one 30 years old, from the United States, single and from a large Irish family, and another, 47 years old, married with four children and also from a close family. At our first face-to-face meeting, we spoke for hours. As I have said before, there are some things you just cannot talk about with your family. I know this and he knew it, as well. He called me an angel that was delivered to help him through this event in his life. I am not sure about that, but he was correct that we shared a lot in common. Perhaps it was to take my mind off my own problems by helping someone else with theirs.

Over the next couple of months, I became close to Aroldo, his wife Lydia, his daughter Jennifer, and his son Harold. Jennifer, a young girl, possessed a talent for singing and performing. She had already started receiving awards before I even met her, and she is still moving up talent-wise today.

Harold was having a rough time. I remember having conversations with his wife about the problems with him and his ability to mentally handle his father's illness. This was a tough situation, and I knew how hard this could be on your family because mine had been living with the stress for a year now. The problem was it really was not my business, at least not yet. Aroldo, Lydia, and Jennifer were frequent visitors, as I was to their house, between January and late February. In late February, Aroldo became too ill with his heart failure and was admitted into Allegheny Hahnemann Hospital in Philadelphia to begin the wait for his heart transplant.

I remember, at Lydia's request, having a conversation with Harold. He was truly a nice kid. The problem was he was having difficulty dealing with the possibility of losing his father and not having him around. There was no real support mechanism in place for him. The support I had at New York-Presbyterian Medical Center was second to none. Transplant families were required to attend these weekly support group meetings. Aroldo's family did not receive the same support where he was transplanted. As I have said before, the impact on one's family was far worse than anything I went through. Aroldo was transplanted in Pennsylvania which is where the number one organ procurement/recovery organization (OPO) in the country, called Gift of Life, is located and managed.. One thing I have learned after 24 years is that consent rates are always higher when an OPO has an aggressive public education group led by donor family and recipient volunteer speakers. If you meet/see donor/recipient speakers, you can put a name, a face, and a personality with organ donation and transplantation. This education provides an impetus to discuss organ, eye, and tissue donation with your family which results in higher donor consent rates and shorter waiting times for potential recipients. Aroldo received his heart within a month where I had to wait longer.

Harold struggled emotionally with Aroldo's impending transplant. I took the time to sit down with him to explain what would happen and that alienating his family would be the worst thing he could do. I told him that nobody knew better how this impacted a family than me. He knew that I came from a big Irish family and that we were close, just like his family. He was, quite simply, afraid of losing his father. I told him that he should be aware that the success rate is nearly 85% from the surgery. There was no other option—he could either support his father by being there for his family and letting his father know that he would be there, or he could choose not to deal with it. I remember even today what I said to him. "Let your father concentrate on recovering successfully from his surgery and the wait he will inevitably have to endure. Let him know that he need not worry about his family because no matter what, you will step up to the challenge." Harold did just that and chose not to quit on his father. With my help, he went out and started a full-time job, bought a used car, and really put his life together. He currently works in Princeton, New Jersey, and is finishing college. He is a living example of another positive impact of the transplant experience that has nothing to do with the patient.

Let me elaborate a bit more about the support group mechanisms I was fortunate enough to be exposed to during my transplant experience at Columbia Presbyterian Medical Center (now known as New York-Presbyterian Medical Center). At Columbia, there was a powerful support group called, "A Gift of Life, Heart & Lung Support Group." This group was immensely helpful to me but even more so for my family because I was not a part of them until after my transplant. I had a version of the support group designed especially for patients when I was admitted to the sixth floor at Columbia Presbyterian Medical Center. A Gift of Life educated and explained every aspect of transplantation as it would affect both my family and me. It was remarkable. You see, I have always been fearful of the impact the transplant would have on my family. In the group, they discussed the effects of the medications, including Prednisone, an immunosuppressant medication, and how they would affect my emotional stability. Not that I would become psychotic, but I would go from normal to very emotional in a proverbial heartbeat. I remember going to my first support group downstairs (as we patients called it) and wanting to thank everyone. I spoke one sentence then broke down and cried like a baby in front of the whole group. My tears were followed by my family crying. I concluded this was probably the effect of the Prednisone since this never occurred with me prior unless I experienced the death of a loved one. It was an emotional moment, but a happy emotional moment.

The support group went on to explain all about follow-up care, rejections, the visiting of patients to give them emotional support prior to transplant, the Coronary Care Unit (CCU) where we would be when we recovered, what happens during rejection, etc. Sometimes I think my family came out of the transplant experience even more educated than me. It's ironic how things work, isn't it? By the time I was admitted and received the heart transplant, my family and I felt more prepared.

6

Entering The Hospital

From Pete's Journal - Thursday, April 16, 1997 - 11:45 a.m.

"Today, and for the last few days, I developed a persistent cough and went to see Drs. Kossow and Amendo. They heard fluid in my lungs and consulted with Dr. Mancini. When Dr. Kossow returned, she said that Dr. Mancini wanted to talk to me. Dr. Mancini said, "Pete, I think it's time we bring you into the hospital to wait and elevate you to Status 1 on the UNOS waiting list." To say I was shocked would be an understatement! But Dr. Mancini saved my life, placed me on the transplant list, and I trusted her implicitly. So on April 16, 1997, I began my five-month hospital admission.

This morning I spoke to Mom and Dad. They have been troopers. Sometimes I get upset thinking about how upset this is making Mom. If there ever comes a time that you are reading this, Mom, I love you very much. Dad hides his concern well when he comes up, but I know deep down inside this is tearing him up, too. If you ever read this, Dad, I love you equally as much.

My sister, Kerry, went into labor early and had my nephew Brennan who was born premature and struggled to breathe. As I waited for a heart transplant, Kerry's son fought for his life at the Neonatal Intensive Care Unit at Newark Beth Israel Hospital in New Jersey.

God worked in mysterious ways today, as well. Kerry came to visit me when a heavyset African American woman approached her first and ended up speaking to her, my mom, and my Aunt Mil. Now, this is going to sound spooky, but my Uncle Joe, who was Aunt Mil's husband, had passed away the year before. This woman asked about Brennan and said, "Do you believe in God?"

They responded, "Yes."

The woman said, "Then trust in God. Joe's with him and looking after him. Trust in God?" There is not a chance this woman knew about Uncle Joe. I will have a similar event three months later at my hospital that I will share later.

Well, I expected to have a roommate and was pleasantly surprised to find, at least for now, I have my own private room. The TV and phone service are expensive these days. Expensive to the tune of $240 a month. I hope I am not here long. I do not think I can afford it!!

My first day in the hospital is over!"

Friday, April 17, 1997 - 4:57 p.m.

"Trying to get a shower around here is proving to be a problem once again! Fortunately for me, a lot of the people here remember me and made some suggestions on the best times to get a shower and ways to get cleaned up daily.

Today, I had the peripherally inserted central catheter (PICC Line) placed. A PICC line is a form of intravenous access that can be used on a long-term basis or for the administration of substances that should not be done peripherally. It is used for long-term antibiotics, nutrition, medications, or intravenous draws. Deep down, I hope I never have to go through this again. With a little bit of luck, I hope I will be out of the hospital recovered by then.

Tracey and Pat came up late this afternoon for about 3-4 hours. It was fun. They always seem to know how to make me laugh. We work well together with the comedy. We laughed a good portion of the time. She called early this morning and we talked for a while, as well. Tracey told me that Mom is taking this really hard. I do not know what to say to make her feel better. If you should ever read this, Mom, remember, you had **NOTHING** to do with my health. Everything that has happened could have happened to anyone. Do not blame yourself because that would hurt me more than anything else. You and Dad and the whole family have been outstanding through this whole thing. I would have expected nothing less. I love you and light it up!!! (BIG SMILE!!)"

Monday, April 21, 1997 - 1:06 p.m.

"Dr. Robert Micheler, the transplant surgeon at New York-Presbyterian Medical Center who would ultimately perform my heart transplant in August, had a popular news program on ABC entitled *Turning Point*. This was a program comparable to *Dateline* today. Ruth, from Media Relations at New York-Presbyterian Medical Center, called me this morning to request an interview for the following day's program on the subject of Zeno transplant. They were interested in my perspective, as an end-stage heart patient, on whether I would receive an animal heart to save my life. Baboons have similar anatomy structures to humans. My perspective, pragmatically, was if you have a choice between a baboon's heart and death, who in their right mind would choose death? Being in the hospital for over a week, the real benefit from my perspective was a visit from the barber and a hair wash. For those who are wondering why the hair wash is such a big deal, it's because a shower is not the norm in the hospital; it is an exception. This is because you have PICC Lines, IVs, and catheters, etc. that you are not allowed to get wet. Why is this important? As a patient, getting these things wet can lead to infection. As a person awaiting heart transplantation in end-stage heart failure on the UNOS waiting list...an infection means I am immediately off the list until the infection is cleared. This could be weeks and the risk of missing a suitable donor."

Tuesday, April 22, 1997 - 6:30 a.m.

"My sleep was disturbed last night due to hearing 'arrest stat' for a man straight across the hall from me. This is one of the scariest things I remember being alone every night. Will the next stat arrest be my room number?"

Monday, May 5, 1997 - 11:57 a.m.

"On a positive note, the doctor changed my fluid restriction but warned me to take it easy with the fluids because there is still a low sodium concern. No problem here as I complied alright with the 1500 cc restriction."

Wednesday, May 14, 1997 - 5:47 p.m.

"I felt ill the last few days and, as a result, have not written anything. Unfortunately, the physical therapists felt they could loosen 30+ years of tight joints. They were wrong, and it threw my back completely out. Worst pain ever! This time physical therapy (PT) really exacerbated the back pain which returned worse than before. The nurses were able to contact Dr. Bianominovitz (Dr. B.). She prescribed some straight codeine for me which made me sleep; and when you sleep, there is no pain. Boy, did it ever take away the pain! I felt like I was melting into or becoming part of the mattress.

On Tuesday, I went for a chest X-ray. Dr. B. came in to tell me that she had trouble sleeping trying to figure out the cause of my problems. To refresh your memory, this had to do with the stomach and pursuant back problems. Dr. B. said she thought it was one of two possibilities. The first was pneumonia. The second was the possibility of a clot in my left lung that may have already done its damage. Believe it or not, they hoped it would be a slight case of pneumonia. I never thought I would ever hear the day when a doctor told me that pneumonia was the lesser of two evils. As I always say, in a very pessimistic tone, at least I am optimistic!

Both doctors came into the hospital late this afternoon and told me I had pneumonia. Pneumonia can come from not being out of bed enough and because I have been in pain or nauseated the last couple of weeks. The infectious medical team prescribed antibiotics. Dr. B. said it would probably take 2-3 days for it to clear up. Otherwise, if it continues, I will be transferred to the Cardiac Intensive Care Unit (CICU).

I have now launched into my fifth week here in the hospital."

Thursday, May 15, 1997 - 5:56 p.m.

"I had to go through a test today, guess which one? If you guessed to have my PICC Line fixed, you are a winner! This time, I made sure I was more coherent. I made sure they put in three PICC lines because I receive many IVs (intravenous).

This PICC line, as I have discussed before, has been a pain in the neck or upper right chest depending on where they place it. This morning, I woke up with my right shoulder soaked and the catheter leaking.

5:28 p.m. You will never have to guess where I had to go again! If you said, Interventional Radiology (IR) or to have my PICC line fixed, you get the prize.

Anyway, as I was saying, IR came around today and attempted to fix the PICC line again. I think the head of the department made attempts to help me this time. They said that my lines kept forming a sheath around them and blocking up. They said they were going to use a longer PICC line. It backed up on them twice while I was there and that is when I started getting a bit angry. I said, 'Hold it, let's find out why this is backing up right now while I'm still medicated and fix it if there is a problem.' Because the new PICC line is longer, it still seems to be alright. Sitting up also seems to be helping with the gravity."

Tuesday, May 20, 1997 - 4:24 p.m.

"Dr. Mancini and Dr. B. came in with Mary, the transplant coordinator, this morning. She confirmed that I am, in fact, #1 for B+ blood type in the region and the hospital. This is important, you see, because hearts for transplant are matched by blood type, chest cavity size, etc. O universal blood is universal and my type, B+, is a rarer blood type. But this is a positive for me. I can receive either an O universal blood type or my own blood type, B+. That meant, according to the doctors, I am next. I do find that now that I have hit the one-month mark, I am starting to lose my patience. Nagging in the back of my mind, though, I ponder how can I be mad that someone has not died so that I could be transplanted?

I hope my family, especially my mom, understands my irritability and lack of patience."

Tuesday, May 27, 1997 - 10:40 a.m.

"This is the beginning of a good day. I must say a day filled with multiple emotions. Last night, around 10:00 p.m., Hank, another patient awaiting a heart transplant, came in and said that he received a phone call from Jennifer, the transplant coordinator, stating that a heart was available for him.

He asked me to come down and wait with him. I, of course, went and stayed with him until his son arrived. When other patients with whom I have a close relationship, like Al or Hank, receive a heart transplant, I experience a whole gamut of emotions. On one hand, I am happy they received a heart and will soon return to their lives. On the other hand, I find myself a little bit disappointed that it was not me. Every time I feel this way, a wave of guilt comes over me. I know God would not want me to be jealous of others receiving a heart transplant. I hope God will forgive me in the long run for these thoughts. I am not losing faith. I know that soon God will provide me with a heart so I, too, will be able to return to my life."

Thursday, May 29, 1997 - 10:29 p.m.

"I can honestly say that today was a good day right from the start. I slept all the way through the night. The nurses and staff that weigh me came in quickly and together. Then I went back to sleep and would probably have slept until 10:00 a.m. except for the fact that Hank called me at 8:30 a.m.

He sounded fantastic! He was more energetic (three days after the transplant) than I was at 8:30 a.m. He was alert and telling me about what to expect after the transplant. He was planning on being upstairs later in the afternoon. Edna, his wife, came up early in the afternoon and told me he was doing fantastic and shared some of the details about the night before and some of the minimal discomfort he felt. He really demystified the whole process for me. I was not upset about it prior to this, but I am really at ease about it now thanks to Hank. I hope I do as well post-transplant.

Jim and I planned to visit Hank tonight with Dad, who came for the support meeting. One of the nurses came to take us up, but she told us a patient on that floor had a streptococcus infection and advised us not to visit. We both agreed wholeheartedly, and Dad went up alone. Tracey said that Dad thought Hank looked great."

Monday, June 2, 1997 - 9:10 p.m.

"Well, I must say that my day went great today which is always a plus since it's my birthday. As I am sure you are aware, I can think of much better ways to spend my 32nd birthday than sitting in a hospital room and making 20+ people travel over an hour to come and sing "Happy Birthday."

Let me just say who came—Mom, Dad, Gram and Pop Radigan, Gram McGahan, Kerry, Scott and Ryan, Tracey and Pat, Jeanie and Joe, Jen and Jim, Aunt Maureen and Uncle Ed, Uncle Bob and Debbie, Sharon Windisch, Jim Dittmer, and Hank and Edna Dernelle. Funny, I just now counted that 22 people came for my birthday. It is great to have so many people that care so much about me. I must say, I care a lot for them, as well. The events of my birthday visits worked like clockwork since my dad and the social worker coordinated the visit. Security gave us no problem. The nurses were great and very patient (no pun intended).

My phone started ringing early this morning and has been ringing non-stop all day long. It took me until noon before I could get into the bathroom to wash my hair and clean up prior to my birthday celebration. When I went into the bathroom, the phone rang three times, but I let it ring.

The day has been fun overall. God has 2 hours and 45 minutes if he is going to give me his blessing of a new heart tonight for my earthly birthday. However, I continue to have complete and utter faith in God, knowing it will be at His will and time. No matter what, I will not lose faith in Him.

Well, that is all for this year's birthday and today.

Jim, another patient awaiting a heart transplant, is not doing too well today. He feels discouraged because he has been on Status 1 for so long with no movement. I know how he feels. It is so frustrating, and I have been number one for less than two weeks. I pray we both will receive our heart transplants soon."

Saturday, June 14, 1997 - 1:46 p.m.

"Sorry, but yesterday was another bad day for me. The afternoon went downhill fast. When I started to walk any short distances, like to the end of my hall, I started getting dizzy and flushed as if I was going to pass out. Then I had a bowel movement and still felt woozy and flushed. When I walked back to bed, I was completely short of breath. Millet, my nurse, gave me oxygen within five minutes. Dr. Blitzer came in within five minutes after that. He ordered Captopril along with my Lasix. They both can lower blood pressure, but it was already low when I received these doses.

3:45 p.m. Dr. Drusin, who is too quiet, came in this weekend and will begin his rotation today. He appears like he wants to leave as soon as he arrives. That is a pet peeve of mine. Everything turned out okay, but he discontinued the Captopril due to my constant dizziness. Whenever I stand up, my blood pressure drops like a rock, and then I feel woozy like I am going to pass out. Even writing in here is starting to bother me because I have been sitting up to write, thus the woozy feeling. He also told me for the first time to increase my fluid and try to eat more. More fluid? That is a switch for a change!"

Note: At this point, Pete took a fifteen-day lapse from submitting to his journal. He picked up at the end of June as he was moved to the Coronary Intensive Care Unit (CICU) for 15 days.

Sunday, June 29, 1997 - 10:32 a.m.

"Since my health went haywire for a short time, I did not write for the past 15 days. My blood pressure became unstable and dropped at one point to 50/30, and I struggled with shortness of breath, which was not good. This occurred late Sunday, the 14th of June.

To my surprise, Dr. Drusin and Dr. Blitzer, the doctors on duty that week, sent me down to CCU (Coronary Care Unit). What a fiasco. The staff told me I had too many belongings in my room. My mom and Gram McGahan, 88 years old, came to visit and packed up my belongings from my previous room to take them home. She also had to assist Gram McGahan. The amusing part of the whole thing, which I found out later when I was in CCU, was that Greg, a nurse, had given my Mom a gurney to carry the three heaping bags of belongings to the car. With Gram in tow, she barreled around the corner and started to lose control of the gurney as she came around the corner. When she did, she smacked Mrs. Henderson, the most serious nurse ever, right in the rear end and sent her through nurses cart and nearly into the wall. She said she thought the nurse was going to kill her.

It took the doctors about three to four days to stabilize my blood pressure. While all this was happening, I had trouble urinating. The urologist inserted a urinary catheter into my bladder to assist me. After they controlled the blood pressure, my fever spiked. They kept me in CCU until Sunday when my fever broke and then brought me upstairs to a double room in 6 Hudson North. I felt angry,at first because the nurse I knew well, Greg, had promised to get me a single room which did not occur. They removed my urinary catheter for eight hours, but I still could not urinate on my own. To my discomfort, they inserted another urinary catheter for three days before attempting to remove it again. There is nothing worse than a doctor putting a urinary catheter in your penis. Thinking about it still makes me shiver. Famous words from the doctor as he is about to ram a wire up my penis…"Okay, just relax." Seriously!

I said, "Let me do it to you, and you relax!" LOL. Thank God I started urinating on my own and have been since.

In addition to that, Greg came through with a single room for me in 6 Hudson South. Room 255, across the hall from where I was before.

For the past three days, I have been having episodes of heart arrhythmia, which are irregular heartbeats, lasting for more than 10 minutes at a time. The first one on Thursday subsided on its own after about 12 minutes. Friday's episode did not end, and they prescribed Denison IV which slowed my heart rate down immediately. Today, Dr. Chen came and firmly pressed my jugular vein almost to the point of choking me. This is a method, without prescribing medication, to convert back to a normal heartbeat. The episode ended. It is called the Valsalva technique and sometimes works.

The doctors prescribed Calan 40 mg three times a day to assist in preventing any more arrhythmias. I took this medication before, but it was discontinued about a month and a half ago. Dealing with these multiple issues, I continued to pray for a heart before it is too late for me.

I predicted I will receive a heart transplant within the next week and will be discharged home by the 15th of July. I hope God allows this wish and ends my present ordeal."

Tuesday, July 1, 1997 - 3:44 p.m.

"What a frustrating feeling it was this morning. It is hard to explain. Even though I trust God, through faith, I sometimes falter and become frustrated at times trying to understand why God chooses for us to go down certain paths at different times. It has been such a long time now that I have been waiting for a new heart. I have plans I want to accomplish, including helping others for the rest of my life here on Earth. That sounds kind of funny in a way when I say, 'Here on Earth.' I mean while God chooses for me to be here accomplishing whatever His path chooses. I hope He soon hears the many prayers that others and myself have offered up, and I receive a new heart very soon so I can move on with my life. Well, enough with feeling sorry for myself."

Thursday, July 3, 1997 - 6:00 p.m.

"I felt terrible last night and when I woke up this morning. I hate to say this because as much as I liked Pat's pizza, I believe it just killed my stomach last night and this morning. Finally, after two doses of Maalox, it started to feel better. However, I missed breakfast and lunch because I could not eat. Thank God that Dad brought up some of Mom's homemade chicken soup and chicken and rice with sauce.

Dr. Mancini came in early this morning. Everything checked out except for my memory again. I forgot to tell her something important, and now she is gone for the weekend. I was, at different points last night, a little bit short of breath with my bed all the way down. On the positive side (I think!), she told me a heart was available last night, but it came from an older man and was rejected. On one hand, I am glad it was available because it proves to me that I am still being considered; but on the other hand, it is still no heart. I really think I am going to lose it if I do not receive a heart this weekend. I pray to God, if it is His will, for me to receive the heart transplant this weekend. Otherwise, I request God be present when I start to lose it on Monday again.

I felt bad for Dad because he really likes getting up here for these support meetings, and they really seem to make him comfortable with everything that is going to happen. He became stuck in some killer Fourth of July traffic on the way up. I think it took him over two hours to arrive today. He planned to attend the meeting which started at 4:00 p.m. but did not arrive until after 5:00 p.m. I am glad they did not start the tours of the recovery room because he really wanted to see the recovery room. A recovery room is where patients are closely monitored post-operatively. Luckily, because they were sending the tours up in shifts, he was able to attend. He even had time to visit me before his tour began.

Well, that is all for today. I will write again tomorrow unless I am in surgery. I wonder if the computer can send a prayer!"

Friday, July 4, 1997 - 2:09 p.m.

"We are all set for the Fourth of July fireworks that Macy's arranges on the east side of Manhattan. We have been informed by the staff of the hospital that we can see the entire main fireworks display from the south side solarium. Believe it or not, Patient Relations has given us a cable-ready TV for which Dad brought up about 50 feet of cable. The TV service took the cable and connected the TV in the solarium yesterday. This way just in case we cannot see it, we will have the 19" color TV as a backup. In addition, we can see the small beginning display which we would not be able to see from the window.   -

I must say, however, despite all the possibilities for seeing the fireworks display, I would not lose sleep if I were in surgery instead of being here."

Sunday, July 6, 1997 - 9:59 a.m.

"Yesterday was kind of a depressing day. I have had so many visitors that I guess yesterday, with everyone down at the New Jersey shore, I started feeling a bit frustrated and maybe even a little bit sorry for myself.

Later in the day, for the first time in months, I cried while watching a movie. This is part of the reason I did not write in the journal. I guess I should explain myself. I was watching a movie on channel 11 called *Class Action* with Gene Hackman about a father who is a lawyer and a daughter who is a lawyer. Anyway, in the early part of the movie, the mother has an aneurysm. When I saw the mother die, I started thinking about what it would be like if my mom was not there for me during this journey. Of course, with my emotional state these days, I lost it and the tears started flowing. That happened a couple of times last night which was my reason for being depressed.

I think and believe my saving grace is that I have complete and utter faith in God that He will bring me through this as soon as possible. I have been praying every night that God and the Blessed Mother Mary will show me the way to complete faith and walk with me, as described in the "Footsteps" poem, until God's will or plan is done and I receive my new heart.

Dad, Mom, and the family called this morning from their shore house and I spoke with everyone. It is hard talking to them because I do not want them to have a bad time while they are at the shore, but we usually have a wonderful time when we are there together. Maybe that is a little pompous of me because they have always been able to have a good time whether I am there or not. Every time they call, I wonder and hope they do not feel the slightest bit guilty (especially Mom and Dad) that they will not be visiting this week.

Unless something outstanding (like a heart) comes up tonight, then there is nothing more to say today. I will write again tomorrow..."

Monday, July 7, 1997 - 4:18 p.m.

"We went through another major holiday weekend with no hearts for transplant. How frustrating!! I cannot even begin to explain how hard this wait is on patients. When you are a B-Blood Type and you are told on admission that, on average, you should receive a heart transplant within 6-9 weeks, it is discouraging when it is 11 weeks so far, especially when you are number one on the transplant list. I have been number one on the transplant list for five of those weeks which is **EXTREMELY frustrating.** Oh well, enough feeling sorry for myself—I will move on.

I felt bad after Dr. Mancini left this morning from my room. I kind of laced into her a little bit about why is it possible that there can be 6 A-Blood Type, 5 B-Blood Type, and 4 O-Blood Type heart transplants in Allegheny Hahnemann Hospital in the Philadelphia Region, as compared to our four transplants over a 16-week period? Her answer did not make me all too happy either, but I know deep down it is not her fault. She said that Kidney-1, which is the donor awareness program in the Philadelphia Region, is extremely aggressive about promoting organ donation and awareness, which usually lessens the time recipients need to wait for organs. She went on to state they are well organized, which made me angry. She said the counterpart to Kidney-1 here in the New York Region was not as aggressive or organized in educating the public, thus those waiting for organs wait longer. I do not understand how the medical community and patients in this region can allow this lackadaisical attitude. Do they not understand the difficulty potential heart recipients and myself experience? At the end of her visit, I felt bad because I was on the verge of tears, and it appeared as though she was, too. I know she is equally as frustrated with this whole situation. I just left Dr. Mancini a voicemail message saying basically, thank you for listening, and I know you are frustrated, as well.

Apparently, I made a mistake with my cousin, Lynne McGahan, yesterday morning when we spoke; and I shared with her that if I did not receive a heart this weekend that I would really be losing it on Monday. She and her sister (my cousin) Sharon spread the word like rapid-fire that I was losing it (kind of coming unglued). Aunt Mil and my cousin Kathy came to visit this morning with cousin Kathy Bussey's father-in-law, Bob Bussey. My cousin Sharon plans to visit me tonight. If I know my cousin Sharon, I will have a visitor every day this week or she will start tearing off heads or visit herself, even if it kills her. She continues to be a Godsend during this whole medical situation with me."

Wednesday, July 9, 1997 - 9:28 a.m.

"Boy, was I in a wacky mood yesterday. It started out a little bit slow. I feel bad for my father. I feel bad for my whole family because I know how hard it is for my family to wait as much as it is for me. Dad, however, sounds tired when I talk to him. I am worried this is taking its toll on him and may soon endanger his health. Tracey and Pat shared with me last week that Dad looked tired, which is similar to the way I felt when I spoke with him. I wonder if it is in some way my fault for the mellow attitude I have had on the phone when I talked to them recently. I feel bad for the attitude I expressed. I realized I needed to keep my spirits high when I speak to them on the telephone even if I am not doing well.

Greg, my nurse, told me that I can take a shower today. This will be my first time taking a shower in 11 weeks. I am waiting to see Doctor Mancini first before I take a shower."

Saturday, July 12, 1997 - 4:20 p.m.

"I know, I know, it has been a while. What can I say? Even though I am sitting here in the hospital, I have been busy.

I pretty much came down from my shower high yesterday which was pretty wild. I have not been so wired since I was out of the hospital and/or in one of my moods. It was like I was teaching one of my classes, and they were a quiet class and I was really trying to get them into it, so I was acting off the wall. The funny thing is with the heart the way it is, I was wired for two hours and then laid down for an hour, then I was wired for a couple of hours, etc., etc. It was fun while it lasted. I cannot wait to take a shower on Monday to again have that feeling of rejuvenation you get after a shower.. For those of you saying, "Hey, what's the big deal, it's a shower!"

My answer is simple, "Try going 11 weeks without one and then come talk to me."

Healthwise, I have been having heart arrhythmias for the last three days. This is happening more frequently. Today, I had the longest one yet and it lasted from about 3:05 p.m. to about 3:45 p.m. It doesn't hurt and I am not short of breath or anything, but the medical team must slow the heart rate down when it reaches toward the 150s because it could lead to a more dangerous ventricular fibrillation. The two intern doctors tried to slow it down by pushing on the jugular on my neck, the Valsalva method, which worked the last time, but it failed to work this time. Finally, after almost 45 minutes of experiencing my arrhythmia, a medication provided relief. This is the medicine that stopped it twice before, and it worked virtually right away. It is now 4:20 p.m. and I feel fine, as if nothing happened. The doctors said they planned to talk to Dr. Blood, who is covering for Dr. Mancini this weekend, about increasing the Verapamil to 40 mg four times a day, which should slow the heart to normal.

As these are happening, each time I say a silent prayer that God will give me the strength to carry me until a matching organ donor becomes my life-saving gift of life. The guilt is becoming more pronounced as the days go by. All I can think about is the reality that someone has to die so I can live, which is very hard to live with, so I avoid thinking about it.

Sunday, July 13, 1997 - 4:52 p.m.

"I have known for some time that I planned to use my motivational speaking ability and training skills to promote organ, eye and tissue donation when I recover from my heart transplant. One thing that has troubled me is the lack of focused volunteer training being done teaching donor families and transplant recipients how to put their stories together for public education. The groups in NY and NJ needed this type of help and I had the ability to create the training and support them. I met a man named Frank Bodino who is part of the New Jersey Organ & Tissue Sharing Network in New Jersey (New Jersey's OPO). Frank would eventually become a great friend, support to my family, and the best man in my wedding. I would later discover that this need was nationwide. This became catalyst behind the formation of Transplant Speakers International, Inc."

Tuesday, July 15, 1997 - 8:18 a.m.

"I talked with Dr. Mancini today about the arrhythmias I experienced. I felt 6-7 episodes in the last four days or so. This morning at about 7:50 a.m. I had another one that lasted for almost 50 minutes. The difference between these episodes has been little. However, for the first time today, the arrhythmia felt like it was pounding in my chest. I thought I might become short of breath, except perhaps not needing oxygen.

Dr. Mancini came in today, and I had a couple of zingers, sarcastic comments, to make her laugh again. The first was, 'After transplant, will I need any IVs?' I knew she would say yes, and I said, 'Which vein are they going to use since all of mine are blown?' The second one was not from me, it was from Mom who wanted me to ask if I am still on the list. She did not laugh until she realized I was kidding. I put my hand on her shoulder and said, 'What kind of day would it be if I did not throw a crack or two your way, huh?' With that, she laughed and left."

Saturday, July 19, 1997 - 2:20 p.m.

"The night before last was crazy. This is probably why there was no journal entry yesterday. Tom Weller (another waiting transplant patient) received a call saying a potential heart was available. I was happy for Tom, but I was more worried about Jim Dittmer. Jim had a rough night the night before because mentally he struggled with being in the hospital after 17 weeks. I have only been here 13 weeks and the wait in the hospital, on the same floor and in the same room, caused me to think I am in a self-imposed medical prison. I can certainly relate to him.

Then about 11:30 p.m. that night, Jim woke me up to share that a heart was available from Ohio. I was happy for him. Then I realized I have no more friends left on the floor. If I am here for a while, I am going to start feeling lonely up here by myself. I stayed up with him until about 1:30 a.m. in his room. Lenny (Jim's friend) woke me up at 5:30 a.m. so I could say good luck to Jim.

Lenny has been up four times to update me on Jim's progress. Jim had some problems. First, he popped a stitch inside on the left side of the heart and they had to take him back to surgery. Then last night he returned to surgery for a third time due to bleeding internally. As of this morning, Lenny said he was doing fine. He was not in any pain, and they removed the endotracheal tube.

Last night I fell asleep around 10:00 p.m. without taking the sleeping pill. I woke up at 1:00 a.m. and took the Restoril and slept like a baby the rest of the night. I needed the rest after the restless night with Jim the night before last."

Saturday, July 26, 1997 - 8:29 a.m.

"I feel bad because Jim called this morning at 7:45 a.m. and I happened to be in the bathroom when he left a message on the answering machine. I kind of snapped at him for calling so early in the morning. I hoped he would be aware of the fact that if the phone rings early in the morning, it might be a potential heart. I knew it would not be my parents, therefore, my first assumption was that a heart was available. My patience is wearing very thin. I later found out, after I politely snapped at him, that he called to tell me John Derr received a heart this morning since John had been in CCU for several months.

The new PICC line was placed yesterday. I tell you I could swear they hit a nerve in my shoulder when they did this procedure. When they put the wire in to prepare to place the PICC line, I felt it in my shoulder. The doctor said I should not feel anything where they were inserting the PICC line because there are no nerves in that area. However, I am telling you my shoulder is killing me today and especially last night. The doctor came in this morning and prescribed Extra Strength Tylenol every 4-5 hours instead of every eight hours.

I feel strongly that the nurses should use sterile gloves and a mask when they attempt to inject anything into my PICC line. I was not forceful enough in making sure they followed sterile technique the last 4-5 days which could be the reason an infection developed.

I still have not received the results from the cultures taken about 3:00 p.m. on Thursday; but hopefully, they will be negative. I am hoping Doctor Lee (who is on duty this weekend) will have the results when she comes in to make rounds.

Mom must have called me four times yesterday. She asked me every time if I received the blood culture results. Yet she continued to ask me the same question which felt so frustrating. The fourth time she asked me, I sarcastically laced into her about asking me the same thing and the fact that just because she keeps asking is not going to change the answer. I know deep in my heart her questions are solely because she cares and loves me. However, as time goes on, I am losing the battle with frustration and anger with her and then feeling guilty over my frustration and anger.

4:07 p.m. Dr. Lee came in late this morning. The results of the culture taken from the location of the last PICC line were positive for a staph infection. The blood work also came back positive, but they were unsure of the type of bacteria. The doctors believe it may be the same.

Well, you might ask what does this all mean now? I am glad you asked. (Glad I still have a sense of humor.) Anyway, the bad news is due to the infection results, I am no longer on the internal hospital list and cannot be considered if UNOS is offered a suitable donor by the end of the day. This does not mean I am removed from any national lists or anything outside of Columbia Presbyterian Hospital. It just means if a B+ Blood Type heart comes in tonight, I will not receive the heart. I pray to God that He waits until tomorrow morning before He gives the hospital a B+ heart. The good news is I will return to the list tomorrow morning. There should be no problem because I have been on Vancomycin since Thursday night. With any infection, they only take you off the list for three days or so because you have been prescribed antibiotics. It will be 3½ days tomorrow morning. There would be no danger to me as long as I wait until tomorrow.

News Flash! I think I finally found some way of adhering the PICC sterile bandage that does not rip my skin apart as the current Tegaderm does. The product is called Mefix. The nurse, Roberta, who works in Interventional Radiology (IR) where they place PICC lines, mentioned it and gave me a long strip of it until they could order some on the floor. I cannot believe the nurses here were not aware of it and did not mention it. I can only imagine it is an expensive product and they may not want to order it. Well, I will tell you what. They will now because the other reason my site may have gotten infected is because of open cuts in the skin due to the tape from the Tegaderm and the red dots caused by ripping tape off skin frequently.

I had requested hypoallergenic patches to replace the red dots, and it took almost a month to force them to order them and for me to receive them. When they sent them, there were only six of them. I replaced my four red dot patches with the hypoallergenic ones but only have two replacements. I guess I should order them now."

Sunday, July 27, 1997 - 8:29 p.m.

"I am back! I am back on the list and there were no B+ Blood Type heart transplants last night that caused me to be bypassed while I was off the list. I thank God again for this blessing.

Dr. Lee came in this morning and told me that I was back on the list, and we talked for a while. I found out from Jim when Hank was here that John Derr was only on the list for about 3½ months and he received a heart. John Rudolf was on the list for about 4½ months and he was bypassed for the heart that John received. I told John Rudolf he should talk to Doctor Katz, who is his doctor, and ask him exactly what is going on. Hank made the mistake of telling him he was only waiting for 3½ months on the list and, of course, John Rudolf became angry.

Today marks 100 pages in the journal. If you have been reading this, I hope it has not been too boring for you. With God's blessing, this will be the last entry until either after the transplant or until I get home."

Wednesday, July 30, 1997 - 9:36 p.m.

"I know it has been a while since I wrote in the journal. Several days, in fact. I just have not been into writing in the journal since I felt I repeated the same things.

Today I was in my room with my father. At around 4:30 p.m., believe it or not, the now-famous heart transplant and cardiothoracic surgeon, Dr. Mehmet Oz, entered and said they had a potential organ donor from Brooklyn, New York. I needed to be prepared to receive the heart which would provide the gift of life. At that moment, I simultaneously wanted to cry and jump in the air for joy!!!!. It was finally my time which was the joy. But reality hit me hard! I felt sad because someone had to die so I could live. In the spirit of Complementary Medicine, Dr. Oz asked the kind of music I wanted to play during my transplant surgery. That was easy. I told him, "Easy! Bruce Springsteen's *Born to Run* and *Born in the USA* albums."

I will never forget being wheeled out of my room to pre-op when, to my surprise, the nurses, doctors, security, food service, nursing assistants, residents…everyone gave me a standing ovation. They had become family. Everyone knew my family by face and name and genuinely cared. It was one of the most moving moments I remember about that night. These frontline workers/caregivers are saints and should always receive the same care, respect, dignity, and PAY they deserve.

My dad called my mom and sisters who raced up the New Jersey Turnpike at 6:30 p.m. My mom was working at JCPenney's and met my sisters. A state trooper pulled my sister Kerry over for speeding. Once the state trooper heard their story, he provided a police escort to the hospital.

I wanted everyone in my family to have zero doubt that I would come out great from the transplant. My energy was super high. Transparent to them, I had recorded a message to each one of my sisters and my mom and dad. Right after we said our temporary goodbyes, I called my father over and said I am not dying; but (I handed him a micro recording device), after I am in surgery, please honor this request and play this for everyone." Begrudgingly, my father agreed, and I entered the surgical suite for a heart transplant saving my life and giving me a new lease on life.

They placed me on the operating table with IVs attached and telling jokes to the staff when a doctor came in and said, "Pete, we are very sorry, but the heart is not suitable, so you will not be transplanted tonight."

I came out feeling sorry for myself until I saw my entire family trying to be brave but with tears in their eyes. I had about 10-15 seconds of self-pity until I saw their faces; and I said, "Hey, I am close to getting a heart transplant. Pizza night!" As if this would make anyone feel better.

It was with profound clarity I realized that what I was going through was cut and dry. I would either live or die from the surgery, but with little or no pain. My family, however, had to watch their son and brother wither away before their eyes. They felt powerless and could do nothing about it.

Still, the reality was never further away than a side glance. The first potential heart turned out to be a bad match, and the news of a no-transplant, which came while I was being prepped for surgery, sent my family reeling into a state of despondency. But the Radigans retained hope."

Tracey remembered the first dose of good news. She admired the capability and confidence of the medical staff and knew Pete was in great hands.

"When we received the first call after waiting for months, that a heart was available, we gave Pete hugs and kisses, wishing him luck, and we could not wait to see him when he woke up."

Anxiously waiting to hear how the surgery went, we find out Pete had been prepped and ready to go for surgery, but they rejected the heart and he had to remain on the waiting list for a new one. No doubt extreme emotions were flying for everyone.

"My youngest sister, Jennifer, echoed this sentiment. 'I remember waiting for months that a heart would be available, as my cousins and family helped care for him and kept him company. When we got word of the first heart, we waited until he was prepped, and then they said the heart had failed.'

Hope faded to desperation. It was back to square one, and time was running out.

My parting thought on this entry is how can anyone not be an organ donor if they think if their mother, father, sister, brother, or close friend needed a transplant? What would they do? Would they let them die or accept a transplant? So again, how could anyone say no to organ, tissue, or eye donation?"

7

The Miracle Of August

(Pete began attending support meetings where he could connect with others going through the same challenges. It was a comfort to be able to share his story among those who had similar experiences.)

This is the life of a transplant candidate. One aims to keep high hopes for a successful outcome, but sometimes it is all about being a number on the list—one that goes up but sometimes comes back down.

The uncertainty of the situation was the reason for the support meetings. Once a week, I would meet other heart transplant recipients, as well as other patients who were waiting for their miracle. The meetings were open to all patients and family members. They would share their experiences which initially started with a subject at hand, such as medicine or therapy. By the second half of the meetings, all topics were up for grabs, and it was rare for a gathering to break up within two hours of its start.

By 1997, Frank Bodino was already a friend of Pete's. They had met at a meeting where Frank shared his story, which was long and grueling, but also successful. Since Bodino, roughly 18 years Pete's senior, received a new heart, Mickey and Ellen Radigan asked Frank to visit Pete in his room, and Bodino obliged.

"Pete was never at a loss for words," recalled Bodino, who quickly bonded with Pete. Although Bodino had already received his heart, he attended the meetings to support the patients who were about to receive theirs.

A lot of the trials and tribulations which stunted Pete's progress had already happened to Frank—the promise of having a potential heart for transplant, introduced by Dr. Oz.

"The same thing happened to me," said Bodino. "It is not uncommon." He went on to add that a donor heart became available the following week. As it turned out, that experience would mirror the events on the grand timeline of saving Pete's life.

But it was more than the shared experiences that drew Frank to Pete. They talked about anything and everything. Frank would wheel Pete to the meetings, and Pete would share about his job.

"He was an ambitious guy," recalled Bodino, whose role as Pete's transplant mentor and confidant remains steady today.

It was the gift of gab that brought the two together to their postoperative endeavor; but in early August 1997, Pete was about to begin the fight of his life. And the thought of what might lie ahead had already ingrained itself into the Radigan family mindset.

As sister Kerry recalls, "When he was waiting for a heart to become available, it became a very real possibility that he may have to take an alternative route if things progressed and a heart was nowhere to be found. They discussed the possibility of transferring a baboon's heart into my brother's body."

Indeed, one of the focal points of the Turning Point piece was the novelty of replacing Pete's weak heart with an animal heart.
But as in many cases during the ordeal, the Radigan's could always rely on their sense of humor.

"My parents and I were interviewed for the show and were asked a lot of questions. It was not until after the show that we noticed the big bar that was right behind us. Nothing like talking about a baboon heart transplant in front of a whole row of hard liquor!"

Pete's recollection of the events of August 1-5, 1997, was a roller coaster of trials, tribulations, and emotions. These are the raw events and anecdotes for Pete and his family leading up to his heart transplant.

Saturday, August 2, 1997 - 12:46 p.m.

"It has been two days after the now-infamous false alarm transplant night. It has been quiet (i.e. no transplants) since that night. Dr. Mancini is on call this weekend, and she remains optimistic that a heart will be available soon. Yesterday she said for the first time, 'This weekend.' She has never said anything like that. No, I do not think she has any insight into the matter; but if she does, let it go from her mouth to God's ears. I think the impact of the false alarm hit home for me and everyone else yesterday. I was physically exhausted and though I wanted to sleep, I could not; but the following night, I slept like a baby. I was out like a light at around 10:30 p.m. and did not wake up until 6:30 when they woke me up for the morning meds. They did not make my bed till mid-morning which gave me the opportunity to fall back asleep off and on for about 2½ hours until Mom awakened me at 9:00 a.m. with a phone call. By that time, I was totally rested. I think I probably could have slept another couple of hours, but it was time to get up as Tracey planned to visit."

Sunday, August 3, 1997 - 7:54 p.m.

"Another weekend has passed and still no word on a possible heart. Nothing since the now infamous false alarm night last Thursday night. It was difficult for Dr. Mancini since she wanted to be optimistic, even for her. Frustration was evident in her eyes. I believe this is the roughest part of the path God has chosen for me to follow for the rest of my life here on Earth. I pray God will end the suffering He has chosen for me soon. It is now taking a toll on my family. It becomes a definite challenge for everyone visiting me. I really hope it ends soon for their sake, as well. The prayer I just said about sums up the way I feel after this long and grueling wait. 'Dear God, into your hands I commend my body, mind, and soul. Your will has taken me down this path, but God, I no longer have the strength. I beg of you, O God, please either save me because you have more work for me to do or take me home. But please, I beg of you to make a decision soon. Into your hands, Lord. Amen!'

Well, that is all for today, I will write again over the next few days unless I go in for the surgery. That would be nice, wouldn't it???"

Sunday, August 4, 1997 - 6:30 p.m.

"I was starting to feel sorry for myself again thinking a new heart might never come. I felt both ashamed and hopeful at the same time. Ashamed times two because I hope someone is going to die and hopeful that if someone died, their family knew of the lifesaving gift organ donation brings so I could receive the gift of life. I felt guilty and selfish for these thoughts.

I received a call from Mary Donovan, the transplant nurse practitioner at about 7:15 p.m. I remember joking with her that she was working so late when she cut me off abruptly, even for her, and said, 'Pete, we think we have found a suitable donor. I will call you back,' and she hung up.

I was like, 'Did I just hear that?'

I called my family and prepared them yet again to come and send me off with their prayers. Once again, I received the lineup from the staff and good luck from my medical team and other workers, etc.

11:00 p.m. I had a much more subdued send-off from my family this time, but everyone felt hopeful that the false alarms were history. The previous trauma had everyone cautiously optimistic since they did not want to be disappointed or get their hopes up again.

My family and I said our goodbyes and made sure we included 'see you soon.' There was no recording because we had said it all during the false alarm the week before. With that, they wheeled me to the OR for the beginning of a two-hour wait for the transplant surgery to begin. Remember, the donor heart and other organs from Tom needed to travel from Buffalo to New York City.

It is said that God is present when there are two or more people praying in a room. God was truly present on August 5, 1997, in the OR waiting room when two other families met and formed a bond resulting from similarities of circumstance. Joe Guidice had been told about the availability of a lung and was waiting. John had been notified of his potential lung, as well. The bond was formed that night when a merciful God saved Joe, John, and my life. The families that endured months or years of suffering watching their loved ones deteriorate had their faith rewarded. The nurse took me to the OR for the transplant surgery."

Monday, August 5, 1:15 a.m.

"All IVs and arterial lines were connected, and everyone was hopeful. I know this is going to sound cavalier, but it never entered my mind that I would not survive. Either I would live or die, but that was in God's hands now. I had really taken to the three main Catholic prayers, The Our Father, Hail Mary, and the Glory Be, and a prayer of thanks for the family that had suffered such loss this same night, when I can celebrate life. I felt exhausted and my mind was really at ease so...I promptly fell sound asleep in pre-op, not from any anesthesia (that came later). I fell asleep because I was tired.

5:00 a.m. But after six hours of successful surgery, the very good-looking Dr. Micheler left the operating room to talk with my family. When he came out, my sisters and mom were drooling because he was so good-looking."

Ellen recollected how her daughters would fight for Dr. Michler's attention. 'It was kind of a joke. He was a good-looking man. Let's not underestimate him. Even though it was not a funny time, it helped us cope.'

Pete's sister, Tracey Radigan (Sabino), agreed. 'Yes!!! Dr. Michler. We all wanted to be the first one for him to talk to! He was very handsome.'

"My dad took notes regarding the doctor's words, which stated that 'The surgery went fantastic. The heart was a perfect match.' There was a collective sense of relief among the family that their son's life was saved. His mother would later state that the medical team said it was one of the best hearts they had recovered. God granted their son and brother a second chance at life. They were all keenly aware that this gift came at a grave price for another family that they may never meet but to whom they would be eternally grateful."

8

A New Life

(After his month-long ordeal, Pete Radigan was ready to chronicle the experience, at least as he remembered it.)

August 6-September 2, 1997

"Well, the transplant went well. Dr. Micheler said the heart was a perfect fit and started right up. The following recap is a compilation of my father's detailed notes and my interviews with nurses and staff.

After the successful transplant, usually within hours, the nursing staff in ICU have us sitting in a chair where they clap you on the back to bring up any leftover anesthesia. They helped me into a chair and clapped me, as well. Some backstory...when you have a heart transplant and they take out your old, enlarged heart, they leave a small piece of your old heart to graft on to the new heart. Now, as I was saying, before they clapped me to bring up the anesthesia, one of the stitches in the graft popped open and I started to crash.

The surgeons came, I returned to surgery, and the popped stitch was repaired. Then five days later, fluid gathered under my new heart and nearly killed me. Dr. Slater went in, made an educated guess, drained the fluid underneath my new heart, and saved my life. As a result of all the narcotics from these three surgeries, over the next week, I felt trapped inside my body which deserves an explanation.

Narcotics, if used correctly, are a good drug to manage pain. Because I was in surgery three times within a week, I was sleepy and could not open my eyes. At times, however, I was aware of people talking in my room and I knew who they were. I just could not open my eyes.

A few stories to illustrate the hallucinogenic nature of narcotics. During the transplant, I distinctly remember hearing, 'Do you believe the heart has been out for 10 minutes and it's still beating?' I later asked Dr. Micheler and his face blanked, then he said, 'I don't think so.' His face, however, told me the truth. Remember when I said I popped a suture? Well, I was not awake, but in the blackness, with my eyes closed, I could see spurting red.

Before I tell you the next story, I have some pre-surgery advice for everyone. Don't read Tom Clancy terrorist books prior to surgery. Not a good combination when hallucination is a possibility. For about what felt like a week, I felt trapped in my body. I could hear my family talking, but I could not talk. I felt frustrated. Back to my Tom Clancy reference. At this point, I started hallucinating. There was a popup metal trash can outside of my room. When it opened and shut, it sounded like a shotgun blast. I felt convinced the doctors and nurses were terrorists, one by one killing my family as they came to visit, as I cried every night right after they left. When I finally woke up, I was ready to kill the staff for killing my family. My sisters later told me as they were leaving, I would tell them not to go to the right when leaving my room, where they could get killed. BOOM! Of course, they knew I was out of it. Once I woke up, I wanted to kill every doctor, nurse, and these caregivers who I previously thought were saints.

When you are under the influence of narcotics that long, it is easy to lose track of reality. I remember a nice male nurse who planned to give me a sponge bath while in CCU. I thought he was a terrorist desiring to kill my family, and I wanted to hurt him, so I waited to strike. As he attempted to wash my face with a washcloth, I almost bit his finger off. Of course, that ended the sponge bath.

Over the next week, I stabilized and they prepared me to move to the stepdown unit where heart monitoring would continue, which provided me more independence, before going to a medical-surgical floor.

As I recovered in CCU, the staff checked my mental status often, which included day, time, place, and person. This drove me crazy probably due to my previous hallucinations including the terrorist scene. Enter my oldest sister Kerry, ever the sarcastic, comedian sister. I said, 'Please, please, please tell me what day it is?' Kerry was trying to cheer me up, but her joke lost its luster.

She said, 'August 23rd, 2030.' I cried. I thought I'd lost 30 years. I still harass her about that to this day. Do not worry, I still love you, Kerry.

On that note, on to step down and goodbye CCU."

Week Before Rehabilitation

"The net effect of the narcotics and the hallucinations caused me to become paranoid, fearful of taking further opioid pain medication when I experienced pain. I remember crying with my dad in step-down and telling him I did not want to go to the psych ward because I was crazy from hallucinations. My dad said, 'Pete, I need you to trust me on this. It's different, you won't hallucinate, I promise.' I trusted him and took pain medicine and had the best sleep since my transplant.

The next morning is the story that will make you believe in God if you do not already. Remember earlier I talked about my nephew Brennan being born prematurely? I mentioned the heavy-set African-American woman who asked my sister, mom, and Aunt Mil, 'Do you believe in God?' and my family members said, 'Yes.' Then she said, 'Have faith, God will take care of him.' He improved within days and was released.

Fast forward to the first morning in step down. A thin African American woman came into my step-down room and said, 'Would you like a prayer?' Always open to a prayer after a transplant, I said, 'Yes.' She then grabbed my shoulders, shook me, and yelled, 'Be GONE…Be GONE, God bless you.' and left.

I was still marveling at what happened when my good friend, Sandy from Food Service, came in two minutes later. I told her what happened and within three minutes she was out investigating. What she said when she returned astonished me, and I have faith and believe in God. She said no one ever saw the lady or anyone that remotely looked like the woman, and I did not hallucinate and was not sleeping when Sandy walked in.

All I can say is God works in truly mysterious ways. I should be happy now. Nope, for the better part of the time leading into rehab, I felt depressed. After spending under five months in the hospital, the medical team informed me another five months would be spent in rehab. This was hard for me because I just wanted to go home. My parents, however, were older and unable to care for a grown man whose legs did not function well. It was unfair of me to even ask, so off I went to in-patient rehab. Healthy + rehab = go home was okay except for the depression around being healthy but unable to go home. I was snapped out of it by the most unlikely of good friends."

Wednesday, September 3, 1997

"I was still bummed out and feeling sorry for myself. I was discharged from Columbia Presbyterian Hospital and transferred directly to their in-house rehabilitation wing. They told me I would have to wait three weeks until space freed up, which made me angry that I would have to wait that long. I was already upset that I had been in the hospital for almost five months and now needed to wait three weeks to start and then do rehab for another 4-6 months. I felt bad but I needed a favor from Dr. Micheler. Since I did some media for him previously, I needed a return favor. I requested that he try to admit me to rehab sooner than they stated. I think back to the audacity I expressed, but I felt desperate. I am still ashamed of my behavior today. I did call him when I was being discharged from rehab and sincerely apologized for my behavior."

Friday, September 5, 1997

"I have now been in rehab for two days and not much has changed. I observed a lot of people with prosthetics who were learning to use them, and believe it or not, still feeling depressed or just generally bummed out. That is when my good friend, Don Arthur, came to visit.

Let me tell you a bit about Don, the nicest, caring human being ever! Ten months after his life-saving heart transplant, Don race-walked the New York Marathon with the Road-Runner Club in New York. That September, he wore a band with my name on it to remind others to pray for me. This very morning Don walked in to give me a pep talk. When he heard me feeling sorry for myself, he said, 'You are selfish!! Look around you. Do you see other people around you without limbs learning to walk again? Are they complaining? YOU SELFISH BASTARD!' With that, he walked out of the room, and I did not see him again for two days.

Don, my friend, did not sugarcoat it. He tells it like it is, and Don was right. It was the call to action I needed and would set the tone for my return to work a mere three months later full time. When Don left that day, I asked my father to stop and get me 5 lb. ankle weights. I told him I planned to sleep with them and wear them during Physical and Occupational Therapies. My motivation included my tenacity, the ankle weights, and two of the best-looking physical and occupational therapists I have ever seen. I would have exceeded anything if only to just impress them.

They said in 3-6 months I would walk out with a walker, and I walked out with a cane three weeks later!

Here is how it happened…"

Saturday, September 6, 1997 - 9:02 a.m.

"I finished my first three days of rehabilitation making good progress. Coming out of the hospital, you need to remember that because of the transplant and two subsequent surgeries, the muscles in my lower back and legs had atrophied and I could not stand and barely could move in the bed unassisted. Here I was admitted to in-patient therapy to get my legs functioning better and I was thinking, *I don't even know where to start.* On Wednesday after starting my therapy, I could not stand up without the assistance of a raised high-chair. If you are wondering what a high-chair is, it's a chair that electronically lifts you to help you stand up. I knew deep in my heart that if I could just hold my own weight in place, it would truly be the start of my physical recovery. I felt pleased that today I could almost get up from the toilet on my own, unassisted. I hope by next Friday I will be even stronger and able to walk longer distances and manage to get in and out of the car. Pam from Occupational Therapy should be working on that with me early next week in preparation for my day trip home on September 14th. It will be a nice break getting out of here for the day for the first time in almost six months. I still find it hard to believe I have spent six months of my life in the hospital. It felt good to start returning to my previous state of functioning.

When I return on the night of the 14th, I will have two weeks of therapy left before my projected day of discharge. That should be tolerable with the break. I look forward to seeing Brennan Peter at his Christening.

My physical therapist, Maria, pushes me as I push myself. The staff, including Dr. Even, Dr. Bartels, and Dr. Rose, are highly competent in every way and will do everything they can for you. Dr. Bartels has given me access to the nurses' Pentium computer so I can access and surf the internet. I also have free reign of the hospital to visit people and go downstairs to the support meetings on Thursdays.

Last night I felt scared, and due to some changes with burning and blood on urinating, a urine sample was sent to check for infection, but this was short-lived.

I had to make this entry tonight. I finally got up from the toilet on my own, pulled up my pants, and walked back to bed completely unaided. As a matter of fact, the nurses were not even there. I will probably get in trouble for that later, but after this triumph, who cares. I will take the heat. I must now work hard to tone up, get the muscles stronger, and increase my endurance. Endurance is the word of the week next week.

I spoke to Mom to inform her of my progress. I told her that I wanted to be able to walk completely into Brennan's Christening. I cannot wait because I will be that much stronger after a week. Maria, my physical therapist, will kill me when she finds out I walked to the bathroom without assistance, but I will take the heat from her. They are mainly interested in my safety, but I will ask them to authorize me for unassisted movement within the room. More endurance building. I have the 2½ lb. weights in the room and am doing exercises with them twice a day to strengthen them. Any more than that and I might be tired for therapy on Monday. Therefore, I will follow her instructions on this.

12:40 p.m. I felt a bit frustrated today getting out of the wheelchair. Sometimes I can, but other times I fall just short by inches from getting to the point where I can stand up with no problem. I got up from the toilet and left the bathroom on my own unassisted twice today. I do not think that is an issue."

Tuesday, September 9, 1997 - 7:10 a.m.

"What a day yesterday was! I think I shocked the whole rehabilitation staff up here with my progress from Friday to Monday.

I can now completely get up from the wheelchair, lowered bed, the toilet, a lower blue chair in occupational therapy, and the mats unassisted. In addition, during physical therapy, I did knee bends (stand straight then bending the knees) and walked from the furthest mat all the way down past the nurse's station, made a left, and walked up to my room at the end of the hall, turned around, and walked back to the nurse's station unassisted and without stopping. I will tell you what. If Maria, the physical therapist, had not stopped me, I probably could have gone much farther. At least back to the mat in the physical therapy room without assistance or stopping. My heart rate and blood pressure were normal when I walked. Pam from occupational therapy encouraged me to get in and out of the Hyundai Sonata car with relative ease. Getting in was no problem. I could not quite manage to get out on my own; but with minimum help, it happened. I predict I will need no support by Wednesday of this week.

Last night was a nightmare. I barely slept at all because of my new roommate. He groaned, spit, called the nurse like every five minutes asking for more water. I ended up putting the TV on just to mute some of the noises.

I spoke to Dr. B. yesterday and just wanted to bust her chops a little bit for not seeing me in a while and almost forgetting her name. Apparently, she has been put on a research project by Dr. Mancini with unbelievable deadlines. I laughed and she said she would visit me soon and would bust my chops right back. I look forward to seeing her, as she is one of the few doctors I know, next to Drs. Kossow and Amendo, who are always upbeat and positive no matter what."

Thursday, September 11, 1997 - 8:26 a.m.

"Yesterday was a crazy day and a good day, therapy-wise. I walked even farther in physical therapy today. I walked from the far mat in physical therapy out and down the hallway, past the nurse's station, hung a left and went to my room, turned around, then continued walking back, stopped while still standing, and talked with Dr. Bartel. I then continued to the nurse's station, hung a right, and went all the way back to the door of physical therapy, hung a left, and went halfway down the hallway to occupational therapy. This was twice as far as I walked two days before. I also got out of the car with just touch assistance. I hope this morning I can get out of the front seat unassisted.

It bothers me a bit that Maria and Pam do not want me to go into the bathroom unsupervised due to the possibility of falling and hurting myself. I had been doing this without their permission and feeling good about it. They will probably give me permission by this weekend.

Sunday, everything is approved for my day pass out of the hospital to go to the Christening. Mom will be up today at 1:30 p.m. to review any tips from the physical therapist for spotting. Then we will be attending the board of directors meeting for the Make-a-Wish Foundation. We will return to occupational therapy at 3:00 p.m. I am excited to attend my second support meeting post-transplant, and Tracey plans on joining me during the latter part of the support meeting."

Friday, September 12, 1997 - 1:54 p.m.

"I thought today was going to start off well, then a complication arose. I knew things were going too smoothly up to this point. It seems that I pulled a tendon just above my left knee cap. It felt a little bit tender this morning; but as I went through physical therapy and occupational therapy, it started to swell up. I iced it a couple of times today already. Sitting and standing from a low position that requires me to bend my knee a lot caused the most pain at this time. Standing and walking do not seem to be a major problem, although it is now swollen.

Physical therapy went well this morning. I walked over 750 feet today. From my room, straight past the first nurse's station, up past the second nurse's station, down to the hallway by occupational therapy, and back to my nurse's station. I made two laps and then halfway back to my room when Maria stopped me. This afternoon, for the first time, I will try the treadmill and continue with climbing the stairs. Yesterday I did all four stairs two-handed up and down while my mom was here. I completed the first two stairs with one rail like it would be at Mom's house. Although it was more difficult, I accomplished both without assistance.

I felt frustrated and slow today in occupational therapy because I could not do the low sit and stand due to my knee problems. Since it may take a few days to heal, I am glad it is the weekend. Hopefully, on Monday, I can pursue it with more intensity.

Finally, today both Maria and Pam gave me the authorization to go to the bathroom without supervision. This is a milestone for me, although I have been doing it for a week.

I felt surprised that Mary Donovan, amidst complaining, completed my long-term disability doctors' portion in record time since I thought it would take longer. I can submit it to Ricoh, my employer, tomorrow.

At my physical therapy session this afternoon, I had a heart-to-heart talk (no pun intended) with Maria, my physical therapist. We talked about my goals and release dates and where the physical/occupational team thought I would be by the middle of next week. We discussed my future functioning at home and the tasks I could accomplish if they discharged me next Thursday or the following week. Even though she felt pleased with my progress, she did not commit herself. She will re-evaluate me on Wednesday next week and will have a better idea. I suggested to her that if I could use the walker independently, it might hasten my discharge and then continue with outpatient therapy at home. However, if they think I may be able to walk unassisted with a cane in another week, I could wait until that time. Since I have been here since the middle of April already, what is another seven days since I continue to progress? I think this is logical, but I will further discuss this with my family for their valuable input."

Monday, September 15, 1997 - 7:43 p.m.

"Sit back because this will probably be a long entry. How exciting for me! Yesterday, I went home for the day pass. It was a glorious day outside. Dad and I got underway home at about 9:45 a.m. and drove straight down to my house where I saw John, Pedro, Fiona and Thomas, Hans and Michele, and Bill and Doreen. I felt so exhilarated to see them! I got out of the car with no problem, and it felt wonderful to walk into my house. It has been a long road, but I cannot wait to be discharged home and move on with my life.

The Christening went well. I walked into the church unaided using a walker as everyone stared at me, which I got over quickly. It felt good to see everyone and be away from the hospital. At one point during the Christening, the priest asked everyone to stand and raise their right hand and pray for the children being baptized. I had been sitting during the entire mass in the wheelchair; but at this point, I locked the wheels, stood up, and raised my right hand to offer the blessing to the kids. When I saw my sister's face, it brought tears to my eyes.

After the Christening at the church, we went to my sister Kerry and my brother-in-law Scott's home to watch some of the Jets and Giants game and wait until the 3:00 p.m. reservation at Basile's Restaurant. The dinner tasted great as I ravaged the pasta and the chicken cutlet parmesan. Mrs. Allmers had made her high cholesterol, high fat, high sodium hors d'oeuvres. I could not eat them, so when I arrived at the restaurant I was starving.

After dinner, we returned to Kerry's house and stayed there and rested, which was about 5:30 p.m. I felt pleased that I functioned well all day walking up steps, inclines, and was able to get in and out of the car unaided. I struggled to get up from the toilet. I could have made it up except I did not want to further injure my strained tendon in my left leg. The second issue was getting in the car again because my knee swelled due to the strained tendon. I solved this by having my dad spot me in the back and I lifted my left leg, balancing with my right leg, and stepped into the car. I did this a few times, unaided, with no problem.

I returned to rehab that night, and the next day was a great day in therapy. I told Maria and Pam about the day out and they were elated at the progress. When I arrived at occupational therapy, Pam observed me getting in and out of the back seat of the Sonata in the O.T. room with no problem. Then we went into the bedroom they have, and I got down on the bed and stood up again with no problem. After that, I went to physical therapy with Maria. I sat on the low mat and got up with no problem. Then I walked on the treadmill for over an 1/8 of a mile. My afternoon session with Maria broke new ground. I went up and down the equivalent of 16 steps (1+ flight of stairs) up and down with two handrails and one handrail. Then I asked Maria if she feels lucky? She asked me why? I told her to give me a cane. She did and I ended walking with a cane back to my room from physical therapy without aid but with Maria at my side and my wheelchair behind me, just in case.

After all of this, the doctors and Maria and Pam decided that I was ready to leave this Thursday instead of the following week. Great news for me and my family. Finally, I will be going home after five months, which was a milestone since I was told it would take much longer.

My gall bladder issues could put a damper on my discharge on Thursday. However, the discomfort has not changed my heart surgery in any way. Dr. Mancini stated that I needed to wait six months when I am stronger, and the surgeon will remove it. The gall bladder surgery is an outpatient surgery and includes anesthesia.

My gout attacks are acting up again, perhaps from taking the Lasix. My left big toe is very sore. Dr. Rowe visited tonight, and we discussed it. She stated she would have to check with the transplant team before prescribing Colchicine. (Actually, that was my idea and she agreed.) Either way, I will be in pain in the morning since the pharmacy is closed, so I hope to receive the medication soon. I plan to contact the transplant team early in the morning if this feels the way I think it will."

Thursday, September 18, 1997 - 7:19 a.m.

"I cannot believe the day has come, but I am being discharged from rehab to go home after five months, six weeks after my heart transplant. I will be discharged around 5:00 p.m. The only reason I am being delayed from 11:00 a.m. to 5:00 p.m. is that Doctor B. wants to review the results of the biopsy. Assuming the biopsy test results are negative, I will be outta here.

It is funny, I would never think I would have been here five months and three days. I look forward to my freedom again. I will have some limitations for a short time because I will not be able to drive, which will decrease my ability to go where I want. It has been a long time, but I am finally going home!

The gout from the other night has disappeared, thanks to the Colchicine medicine. Doctor B. discontinued the Lasix 40 mg so, therefore, I should not need to start taking Colchicine as a preventative medicine. I need to inquire from Dr. Mancini or Doctor B. any directions after discharge which includes my sugar levels, diet, and ability to drive, which should be soon.

Later today I plan to attend the support meeting and will enjoy the pleasure of announcing to the group that I will be going home today. I hoped I could attend the support meeting, but if I were discharged too early, I would not be able to. However, since I was discharged later, I was able to attend.

Well, my next journal entry should be from home..."

PART III

The Path To Healing

9

New Beginnings

*For Pete Radigan, the second chapter of his life was about to begin.
But for Janet Mauk, ambivalent feelings arose. Sad because Tom was gone.
Happy because his wish had been fulfilled. However, the first year after
Tom's death was a difficult time as Janet grappled with the struggle of
believing the unbelievable and missing Tom. Writing continued to be her
cathartic expression. In a mid-August 1997 entry, Janet wrote:*

"The immediate days following the funeral, I fondly and lovingly
wrote thank you notes to family and friends who so kindly
supported me in multiple ways. I thanked the staff and nurses in the
Trauma Intensive Care Unit at Erie County Medical Center
(ECMC) and brought them some candy. I cried myself to sleep
many nights. And yet, I was thankful to be Tom's MOM to love and
care for him for 16 years, 349 days, and 20 hours. I missed him a lot.

My trips to the cemetery have been almost daily as I read the small
marker on his grave which says, 'Thomas Corbin Mauk,' trying to
believe it. I knew he was not there. But just reading the marker
helped to confirm the reality of his death. However, it seemed more

like TOM to be bounding through the house at any time, and saying, "Mom, I'm home!!!" He was so full of life and love. I reviewed the events of the accident often as friends listened with compassion until I could believe it. I found it enjoyable to reminisce with friends about some of Tom's antics, as we laughed and cried because we missed him. Many friends would say, 'I can't imagine losing a child.'"

August 19, 1997

Days later, a somber reminder brought the Mauk family together. Today would have been Tom's 17th birthday. She wrote:

"While having lunch with Tim, some friends had sent me a dozen beautiful red rosebuds to remember Tom's birthday, which brought me to tears. Friends sent me cards every day, with notes reminding me that I believed in Tom and never gave up on him.

I had this compulsion to sit in Tom's bedroom at his father's house, just to be close to his belongings, and after to view the accident scene. As I pulled into the driveway, I wept as I recalled the place Tom stood, nine days before he was killed, which was the last time I saw him alive. I envisioned him in that same spot. Who would have known?

As I went into his room, I saw the little piece of paper on the door which said 'Mom, 3 pm Thursday.' That was the last day we spent together. I viewed the items in his rooms, including his previous Christmas gifts I gave him, reminders of better times.

Then Tom's father, Tim, and I visited the accident scene. After I saw it, I felt so thankful God spared me from finding Tom after the accident in the middle of the road. It had to be horrible. I was thankful he became unconscious quickly following the accident."

"I had thought little about the recipients of the organ, tissue, and eye donation," wrote Janet, just three days after her previous entry. "But today I received a letter from the Upstate New York Transplant Services, Inc. (UNYTS) about whose lives received the gift of life or enhanced through donation by saying yes."

The letter read:

August 22, 1997

Ms. Janet Mauk

189 80th Street

Niagara Falls, NY 14304

Dear Ms. Mauk,

Please accept our sincere condolences over the loss of your son, Thomas. The gift that you have given through donation has permanently changed the lives of transplant recipients and their families. Your concern for others during a time of personal grief is admirable and genuinely appreciated.

A 32-year-old gentleman from the New York City area received a life-saving heart transplant. He is engaged to be married and is looking forward to his upcoming wedding and being able to return to his full-time job.

A 66-year-old male, also from the New York City area, received a life-saving lung transplant. He is recovering well and looks forward to returning home from the hospital and spending time with his family.

A 54-year-old construction worker from Long Island received a life-saving lung transplant. He is recovering very well and is thankful for his second chance at life.

A 51-year-old woman from New York City received a life-saving liver transplant. She is married with two children and expects to be discharged from the hospital soon.

A 39-year-old gentleman from Rochester received a pancreas transplant. He had diabetes and due to his transplant, he will no longer need insulin shots several times daily. He also is experiencing a quick recovery and looks forward to returning home to his family and full-time job.

A 36-year-old woman from Kansas received a kidney transplant. The kidney was a "perfect match" for her, and it is highly unlikely that she will ever experience any type of rejection. She is a college graduate and works full-time at a daycare center. She is now free from the rigors of dialysis.

An 8-year-old boy from Buffalo also received a kidney transplant. He experienced difficulties with dialysis and he and his family are most grateful. He has been discharged from the hospital and is recovering well at home. The bone and tissue will be used in individuals who might have otherwise been permanently disabled. These individuals, many of whom are young children, now have a second chance at experiencing a greater quality of life.

A 36-year-old from Olean received a sight-restoring cornea transplant. The other cornea was transplanted into a 70-year-old from Long Island. Both are doing well at this time.

On behalf of the recipients and Upstate New York Transplant Services Inc (UNYTS), thank you again for your kindness and generosity.

Sincerely,

Cheryl O'Donnell, RN

Organ Services Coordinator

Kevin Gramlich, RN

Organ Services Coordinator

The reason Janet had not thought much about the potential recipients was due to her grief and readjustment after his death. But the letter from UNYTS (now Connect Life) injected her with hope, compassion, and the knowledge that lives had been saved. They could now smile easier, function better, and return to a better quality of life. As she wrote:

"I read the letter and WEPT!! The feelings of intense sadness and joy coexisted. Can gratitude and grief coexist?? Sadness Tom was no longer here, and happiness others could live because of saying yes to donation. SO, for the rest of the day, I contacted friends and family to share this wonderful news—in between tears—as they began to process it as well. I felt thankful God gave me a choice about life for others, on the darkest day of my life."

Even though Tom's shortened life now extended life for others, Janet's friends and family were somewhat befuddled.

"As I shared this letter with others, they asked many questions. Some said, 'How could you make the decision at a time like that being faced with his unexpected death and on the other hand being asked about organ donation all at the same time?' The thinking was: Here you are faced with a tragedy which takes time to absorb, and then ask to donate? It almost seems cruel. I responded by saying that during this entire process I asked the neurosurgeon a lot of questions, and he showed me the results of the MRI. Seeing Tom's cranial fracture further confirmed his poor prognosis. How could I not say yes to donation when his potential death was out of my hands but saying yes could bring life for others?

Others wondered if the medical team would try as hard to save Tom knowing there was a donor shortage. Having worked in nursing most of my life, I felt confident that the physician's role is to provide the best care possible to save lives. Just the fact that the neurosurgeon offered us two options was proof enough for me that the medical team was doing everything possible.

Another question posed was, 'Hasn't Tom already suffered? Why put him through more?' Tom never regained consciousness, his prognosis was poor, and his death was imminent. When procuring the organs, tissues, or eye donation after death, the patient is dead and no longer feels any pain or discomfort. The potential for changing the world at that time is sorely misunderstood.

Another question was, 'How did I know Tom would not recover?' citing others who have recovered usually after a few years but marginally functioning. After working in the field of nursing, I had no doubt making this decision was the right one.

Others stated it must have taken courage to make that decision. I replied, 'It just seemed like the logical decision since Tom loved people. His death was out of my hands, but life for others was in my hands which was a gift in the middle of a tragedy…and not everyone has that choice.'"

Not that Janet's sadness was healed by any means. She attended Compassionate Friends, a support group for those who have lost a child. It brought Janet into contact with people who shared her experience. She explained:

"After listening to the stories of others, it distracted me from my own grief, as I felt thankful my situation was not worse. Then, it was my turn to share my own story. It felt difficult to share, and I became emotional, stopping at times. In the room of at least 40 participants, everyone welcomed tears. There were no adages or advice, but hugs, understanding, silence, and support. As I traveled home, I would listen to Christian gospel music, reminding me of God's sufficiency and presence which soothed my heart and soul.

I attended a four-week presentation on grief at a local church. The facilitator immediately remembered the accident and shared that the EMTs attending to Tom at the accident scene needed debriefing the day after the accident since one worker had a child Tom's age. She normalized our feelings and provided education on what to expect during the grief journey, which was helpful.

One of my joys during my grief was creating a scrapbook of Tom's life through pictures, called creative memories. A dear friend had given me an album with the front page in calligraphy with Tom's name, date of birth, and date of death. It helped me start the healing process as I would place his pictures in the album, even though I started with the most recent memories. I could not look at his baby pictures yet. Some days I would complete several pages and some days I did not do any. This brought a smile to me as I captured through pictures the wonderful memories we shared.

One night as I prepared for bed, I turned the radio on to "Focus on the Family," and the topic was organ donation. The father, who was a physician, and his son's recipient were talking about the value of organ donation. I was moved at hearing this story, though bittersweet, as I cried. His son had suffered a skiing accident and was pronounced dead in the ICU. The father spoke of how difficult it is to let go. After the presentation, I cried myself to sleep.

The following night, they discussed how the recipient and the donor dad met. I cried again, knowing I would not be ready yet to meet any of the recipients, but I knew that Tom would be happy to know he gave life to others."

In January 1998, Janet's friend, Mary Ellen, needed to fulfill her duties in the Army Reserves in Savannah, so she invited her to go along. This would give Jan the chance to visit her older son, Tim, who was still stationed there, and Jim and Gerry, friends she had spent time with the year prior. However, every time Jan thought of returning to Savannah and flying there, she felt overwhelmed with sadness and tears since Tom made the trip with her last year.

"I struggled with stepping on the airplane without Tom. I did not make the decision to go until the night before, praying that God would give me the courage and He did."

What she did not expect was how transformational that step would be. As accounted by Janet:

"After arriving, Tim and I arranged times to visit due to his schedule. I also made time to visit with Jim and Gerry who Tom and I stayed with the previous year. As Jim, Gerry, and I walked in a nearby park, we discussed Tom's accident and death. They said, 'It did not surprise us that you decided to donate his organs.' 'Really?' I surprisingly replied, 'how did you know?'

They continued by sharing that during our visit last year, Tom and Jim stayed up late talking. Tom asked Jim if he had marked the section on his driver's license about donating his organs if he were to die. Jim replied that he had. Tom stated, 'That is what I want to do when I get my license. If anything happens to me, I want to donate my organs to help others.'

Gerry went on to say that Tom brought it up many times the next morning, almost obsessing about it before I awoke. Since Tom felt so adamant about this subject and continued to focus on it, Gerry tried to change the subject.

I had never been privy to this information until that moment. Tom never talked with me about it. I felt thankful for this information; and even though I had no doubt about making the decision to donate, it confirmed to me that Tom had thought this matter through and would make that decision.

Over the past five months, I had occasionally thought and wondered about the recipients, hoping they were doing well. If it worked out, in the future and when I was ready, I looked forward to corresponding with them and perhaps meeting them, if they so desired.

It was both a delightful and sad time to spend time with Tim while in Savannah. We reviewed Tom's accident, and I answered any unanswered medical questions Tim had. We both missed Tom a lot as we reminisced about some of his antics with tears and laughter. We stayed in contact with each other, checking on how we were coping and asking for God's help through our journey."

10

Making Contact

From Janet's Journal - February to March 1998

"Since there had previously not been any witness to the accident, we were never sure of the details. About six months after the accident, a witness came forth to describe the accident. The witness was driving and came upon a well-lit crossroad, slowly thinking he could cross, but looked to the left, and he immediately heard a car driving fast, turning to see a young lady driving with a passenger. Due to her excessive speed, he did not venture forth. She apparently did not see Tom and hit him at the rear of the motorcycle. After she stopped, she got out of the car and walked over to see Tom lying in the road and passed out.

The EMT later stated that Tom's right pupil was fixed and dilated, and the left side of his face was swollen shut. While composing the report, the doctor later wrote impending herniation and brain death. It was stated that even though he had a helmet on, it snapped off. Motorcycle parts were all over the road. The Glasgow Coma Scale (GCS) reading was three at the scene of the accident. (Note: Three is the lowest possible score and is the sum of three factors—eye response, verbal response, and motor response. Scoring a one for each category indicates a deep coma or death.)

Of course, at that time we were not privy to that information. I was again thankful that Tom was taken quickly instead of readjusting to a lesser quality of life with rehab. Also, the driver's insurance adjuster told her not to plead guilty for excessive speed, but she did anyway. When I heard of her honesty in pleading guilty, I felt a lot of respect for her.

Since the accident, the staff at Upstate New York Transplant Services (UNYTS) now Connect Life, showed their support. I would occasionally contact the staff and inquire about the recipients. According to the information they had, the recipients were doing well, which thrilled my heart.. **It was a real sacrifice to donate, but the bittersweet thinking is that I hoped the recipients would remember this sacrifice and take care of these wonderful life-altering gifts.**

UNYTS told me that Tom gave more of his organs and tissues than anyone ever did. The miracle of it all was that, even though his head injury cost his life, there were no other injuries to the rest of his body. After hitting her windshield, he flew over her car, and landed 178 feet from the point of contact, landing on his head. He was a perfect candidate to give everything in donation that could be used to help others. I was thankful we said 'yes' to donation, and only God could have superintended this accident without further injuries so we could donate everything.

The staff from UNYTS informed me that if I wanted to contact any of the recipients, I could send a letter to UNYTS and they would pass it on to the transplant centers. They provided the type of information to place in the letter; however, they warned me to avoid personal information. I assured the staff I was not quite ready yet.

The UNYTS staff encouraged me to volunteer at their facility, which helped me in the healing process. I started by attending a tree-planting ceremony in the spring of 1998 with other donor families in Buffalo. We placed green ribbons on the tree in honor of those who donated. I received a bronze medallion which is shown on the website. I later placed one on Tom's gravestone."

Meanwhile, Janet's concerns about contacting the many people whose lives were renewed by Tom's life-saving gifts were about to dissipate, through no action of her own, as she chronicled in a midsummer journal entry.

Letter from the Heart Recipient, July 28, 1998

"As I went to the mailbox that day, there was an envelope from UNYTS with an enclosed letter from the heart recipient. It was written in October 1997, two months after Pete's heart transplant. I was curious as to why I had not received the letter before. I contacted UNYTS to inquire and was told that the person taking care of the letters left the organization two months ago and they were trying to send out the letters now.

I wept as I read it. I called friends and family to share the wonderful news. They shared my excitement. My tears were happy and sad, happy that Pete was doing well, and sad that Tom was no longer here. It was good timing since I was heading toward the first anniversary of Tom's death.

Last October, I was still in shock, and I didn't want to believe it. The letter went on to say that Pete received Tom's heart on August 5, 1997, and he was in the hospital for another two months.

The letter was full of gratitude. Reading his story made me realize that he would have lost his life if he did not receive a heart transplant. Since I received the letter nine months after he wrote it, I asked UNYTS to check on how he was doing. They replied he was still doing well and checks the New York City office often to see if there is any letter from us. He wants to hear from us. It is as if, after my greatest sorrow, God is there offering joy and making the pain more bearable. I felt motivated to meet him.

I called Tom's father about the letter and inquired how involved he wanted to be at this time. He said, 'I want to let bygones be bygones.' Since I was facing the first anniversary of Tom's death and planning to travel to Columbus for the Transplant Games, I put off writing Pete back until I returned. I also shared the letter with Tim, who missed Tom a lot, wishing he were here.

Here is the letter I received from Pete."

October 13, 1997

Dear Donor Family:

I'm sorry it has taken me a couple of months to write this letter, but I had a few complications related to my old heart that caused me to be in the hospital up until about 10 days ago.

I cannot begin to thank you enough for the gift of life that your son gave to me. I could not fathom the thoughts of losing one of my four sisters or either of my parents. I know that your loss was great, and I pray for God to watch over your family and bless your son every day.

I am a 32-year-old man that has had a heart disease for the past 11 years. In January of 1996, I had right heart failure. My profession is a National Sales Trainer. I was somewhat stable and out of the hospital waiting for a heart organ donor that was suitable. After 1½ years of waiting outside the hospital, my heart failure got worse and I was admitted into Columbia Presbyterian Medical Center where I waited for a heart until the night of August 4, 1997. I was prepped for surgery and received your son's heart on the morning of August 5, 1997. Though I had some difficulties relating to my old heart's enlarged size, I am healthy and strong as I write you this letter. I hope that you can find solace in the fact that your son's ultimate gift has given me a chance after a once uncertain future.

I am actively involved in The Sharing Network in New Jersey to use my speaking ability to promote organ donor awareness so that other people may receive the gift of a future life as I have.

Thank you for my life and I hope that at some point you will make contact with me so I can thank you personally.

Love,

Heart Recipient

At the time, Janet was still not ready to meet the man whose life was saved by her son. Yet she felt compelled to learn more about the transplant community and immerse herself in some of its activities. As the first-year anniversary of Tom's death approached, she decided to mark the occasion in two ways. The first involved submitting a one-year Memoriam to the local newspaper honoring Tom. The second one involved meeting her friend Nancy at the cemetery to share memories of Tom, especially as the clock reached 4:03, the exact time of Tom's accident. She bought some roses and a balloon that read, "I miss you" and took them down to the grave.

"It was obvious at this point that I was being inducted into a new community, one of life and loss, and one that would change my life and change my direction."

1998 Transplant Games and the National Kidney Foundation

"In June, I received literature about the 1998 Transplant Games in Columbus, Ohio, as well as the National Donor Recognition ceremony, and I decided to attend in August, just a week after Tom's first year anniversary. I sent in a picture of Tom that would be shown on a screen during the ceremony. I also needed to make a quilt square to attach during the ceremony. A friend created one for me, of which I felt thankful.

My friend Kathy agreed to attend with me. When we first arrived, we went to the stadium for the opening ceremonies. As we walked in, arriving later than expected, we did not see Tom's picture on the screen. A lady showed it to us later, which brought back happy wonderful memories but also sadness.

The two speakers were Larry Hagman, who received a liver transplant in 1995. The other speaker was Reg Green, the father from the movie *Nicholas' Gift* and his book *The Nicolas Effect*. His son Nicholas was killed while they vacationed in Italy. The parents decided to donate seven organs to save and enhance the lives of others .I then felt moved as the oldest and youngest recipients were introduced to the audience. Knowing Tom's recipients continued to do well returning to their previous way of life, brought me joy.

The next day we attended more seminars related to donor families. The first one was an overview of organ, tissue, and eye donation which was presented by a surgeon. The next seminar was titled "Losing a Child." The speaker had six children and lost her six-year-old daughter from a blood clot to her brain after sending her to school. It was surreal to meet her as she shared her story. She normalized many of our feelings and encouraged us not to allow other people to tell us how to grieve. I also enjoyed meeting other donor families, professionals, and transplant recipients. I met the woman who was in charge of tissue and bone donation. She encouraged me to contact her as she could share with me those patients who were helped by Tom's tissue and bone donation.

I looked forward to the evening session since it involved correspondence between donor families and recipients as they shared their stories, which were moving. Again, I felt thankful my situation was not worse. Twenty-five percent of these individuals lost their loved ones to suicide. As we boarded the bus to return to our motel, organ recipients would come up to me since my name was on my donor family name tag. They could not thank me enough for thinking of others at such a sad time and donating Tom's organs even though they did not know me.

I had many questions answered the next day about brain death during an educational session. A nurse stated the hardest job in nursing was convincing the family their child was brain dead. At the time of Tom's death, with so much swirling in my mind, I did not comprehend it all. I also learned that in New York state, two doctors needed to agree on brain death to pronounce a patient dead caused by trauma, a blood clot, or lack of brain circulation. Friends and families previously raised their fear of donation because they thought the medical profession would pronounce them dead earlier since there was a donor shortage. She said the physicians do not enjoy pronouncing someone dead so they would not rush into it. Also, the medical team does not have any contact with the transplant surgeon at that point.

Next, we attended the Quilt Square Pinning ceremony. Many donor families brought their quilt squares. I pinned Tom's quilt square and shared his story with other donor families who were there. All of us had tears in our eyes as we shared our stories and understood each other's grief.

As we returned home, I felt thankful that I attended. I thought if other donor families could make it through the grief, so could I, even though it sometimes seemed overwhelming.

As I returned from the Transplant Games, I felt energized toward the wonderful opportunity to write back to the heart recipient. I felt pleased to hear the positive stories other donor families who had corresponded with their recipients shared at the Transplant Games. It brought a new excitement. What I did not know was that Karen, the kidney recipient from Kansas, also attended the Transplant Games, unbeknownst to me. Karen sent me a thank you note full of gratitude since she was on the threshold of dialysis. The Hispanic liver recipient from Long Island sent me a letter in Spanish full of gratitude, as well.

So, with caution and not knowing what to expect, I decided to write a letter to Pete."

August 22, 1998

Dear Heart Recipient,

On July 29th, I experienced a sad day in anticipation of the first anniversary of my son Tom's death. The next day, my grief was eased as I received your most welcome, grateful, and empathetic letter, regarding your heart transplant. Your letter must have been detained at the Procurement Office since the time you had written it. When I called them immediately to check on your physical condition, they assured me that you are healthy, and your body is continuing to accept Tom's heart. I admire your courage in writing and appreciate both your condolences and expression of gratitude in receiving Tom's heart.

My son, Tom, was 16, almost 17, and had taken his father's motorcycle out for a drive around 10 PM on August 2, 1997. He was returning slowly towards his residence in the country when a 19-year-old girl, who did not see him, struck him from the rear with her car. He was immediately ejected from the motorcycle, fracturing his skull on her windshield. He lived another 40 hours before respirations ceased. He was pronounced dead due to brain trauma on August 4th, 1997 at 4:03 pm. It is certainly a parent's worst nightmare, and the grief is beyond description. However, I am thankful he did not suffer.

Knowing that Tom's death was imminent, organ donation became a certainty. Six months before he died, Tom told some mutual friends, "If I were to die, I would want to donate my organs so that others could live." Tom's wish came true, and I am thankful that you were able to receive his healthy heart and be given a second chance at life. I am sure the anxiety of wondering and waiting must have been overwhelming for you and your family at times.

I am also thankful that God lent Tom to us to love and nurture for 16 years, 349 days, and 20 hours. We were certainly blessed to have loved him during his time here on earth. I have included a picture of Tom for you. I wanted you to know he was full of love and life and always on the move—socializing with people and charming them with his wit. He was also sensitive, caring, loved animals and the outdoors, and had a perception beyond his years. He truly had a "heart of gold."

It brought me to tears as I read your letter. It was indeed a solace to me. I wanted to write to the organ recipients but thought it best to give myself close to a year, as recommended by the procurement agency, to grieve. Since you received his "heart of gold." I wanted to contact you first.

I am a registered nurse, and my ex-husband works for General Motors. We live in the western New York area. We also have a 21-year-old son who is in the Army utilizing his abilities and interests in aviation mechanics and flying. Though his only brother's death has been difficult for him, I believe the Lord will see him through this difficult time.

I just returned from the National Donor Recognition Ceremony and Workshop in Columbus, Ohio, on August 5-9. It encouraged me to meet other donors and recipients and feel their gratitude during their loss. For this reason, I am also strongly thinking of attending the 48th annual meeting of the National Kidney Foundation in Philadelphia for donor and recipient families.

I trust this letter is an encouragement to you. I hope and anticipate continued correspondence between us.

Love,

Your "donor's Mom," Jan

With the arrival of the letter to Pete, a friendship was forged. Janet found a new purpose in life, and Pete had a name and life history to put behind his new heart. This is noted in their subsequent entries and letters to each other as the details, which would lead to a personal meeting, began to take shape.

A New Focus and Direction, Transitions in Profession

(From Janet's journal)

"After going through the most difficult dark month in August of 1998, the first anniversary of Tom's death, I would never know this major loss could change the direction of my life so much after 25 years of nursing. I always knew I would have a second career but did not know what it would be. Grief caused me to evaluate my life and my role now as I prayed for direction. Do I still have two sons or just one? Am I really doing what I love to do? What is my new direction? One day I realized that I feel fulfilled when I educate and support.

I explored returning to college to obtain a Master's Degree to teach science. But after exploring the requirements and talking with others, I decided to forgo it. A former high school classmate who served on the Board of Education stated, we want the younger teachers and you are older at 47. I laughed, not feeling that old. Tim, my son, a recent highschool graduate, gave me the best advice. He said high schoolers will eat you alive since I am such a nice person. So my attempts at pursuing teaching came to an end.

So I decided to pursue social work.

In July, I matriculated in a one-credit-hour course at the University of Buffalo. I had not attended college in 20 years, so there was much to learn. So much of my energy went into helping Tom, and now I had a hole in my heart and soul that felt empty at times after his death. I felt like a rudderless ship but had faith my purpose would be revealed.

In the fall, as a non-matriculated student, I signed up for a three-hour course in Gender Issues. There were many writing assignments, so I felt challenged at first but found it enjoyable. The UB admissions office felt positive I would be accepted in the Master of Social Work program the following year. I felt ecstatic. I purchased a computer, which I needed, to complete my assignments.

During this time, I also received a phone call from the National Kidney Foundation in New York City, inquiring if I would be interested in becoming a representative from Western New York for the National Family Donor Council, which entailed supporting other donor families which I did accept. A first step toward fulfilling my purpose. I later established relationships with other donor families and provided educational programs for donor families in Western New York, which I found fulfilling.

UNYTS (Connect Life) also contacted me, informing me the letter I wrote to the heart recipient had been forwarded to the NYC office. Pete had received it, but they would not give him the picture of Tom I enclosed because they did not feel he was ready."

Janet was not ready either. In September of 1998, she composed an update that showed her progress through the grieving process but exposed her continuing sense of loss.

The Minor Key of Grief

"September (1998) brought new opportunities, as I felt fulfilled returning to college since I love learning and enjoyed the interactions with other students. It felt like a breath of fresh air. During the first class, each of us had to introduce ourselves and share with the class something about ourselves. I shared about Tom's death and organ donation. My instructor responded by saying, 'There is a gift in every tragedy. I have never forgotten what she said. I already knew what the gift was—organ donation. I would never know at that time how far-reaching it would be. This course and other responsibilities kept me distracted from grief. However, veteran grievers shared that if you are busy or not, when a grief attack occurs, it feels like a tsunami, is exhausting, and slows you down until you recover. At this time in the grief process, friends think you should be over it when, in fact, you have just entered the worst part of the grief the second year. I found that to be true. Some days you think you are alright, and other days you cry buckets of tears. I think all grievers need windshield wipers for their eyes.

The second year found me longing for Tom, wanting to be with him, feeling lonely and empty. I longed for a phone call from him, saying, 'Guess what, ma?' as he would share his adventures. Some days I felt like I was in the emotional intensive care unit, feeling fragile, emotionally vulnerable, mentally disorganized, and not being able to cope as well as previously. The emotional support from others helped to fill that need. Reading the book of Job and other portions of the Bible gave me hope and comfort that I could survive, as well, knowing Job endured multiple losses. It gave me assurance that I, too, could survive by trusting God each day.

I attended a seminar on grief by a professor from the University of Buffalo and learned a lot. He said, 'Sometimes grievers do the strangest things.' Some grievers wear the clothes of their loved one. Sometimes grievers even see the loved one, and others think they are psychotic, but they are not. My need to touch something Tom had touched was normalized, as I held the cloth doll and hand of 'My Buddy,' a large cloth doll Tom enjoyed as a preschooler. It brought me comfort, and I felt closer to Tom. I had previously given the rest of his clothes away.

Friends, neighbors, and relatives continued to ask, 'How do you face the day each morning, knowing Tom is gone?' Several thoughts came to mind. Tom's friend, Craig, and his mother, Nancy, would stop over at times, hug me, and act out some of Tom's body language, sharing good times, which put a smile on my face. Craig told me Tom wanted to surprise me in the future with a GED. WOW! That was so nice to hear. It was a joy to my soul when they would say his name, Tom, in conversations. It was not only a reminder they had not forgotten him, but it also felt comfortable speaking his name. Many people hesitate to name the deceased person, thinking it will bring sadness to the mourners; but I informed them mourners already feel sad, and mentioning their name brings comfort.

Having faith in God, knowing He would be sufficient to meet my needs, feeling confident Tom was safe with God in Heaven, and the support of friends and family propelled me toward healing. I shared with friends and family that I could not and would not give up even though the pain felt brutal at times. Other times, I thought of how to escape the pain. The anesthetic of shock had worn off. I yearned for Tom and wanted to hug him, talk to him, and longed for his presence. It would never be on Earth. When the pain was intense, I thought about running away, moving, or trying drugs to mask the pain. However, I chose to stay the course and depend on God knowing this was His sovereign plan.

Veteran grievers told me you need to feel the feelings as you process the grief, and then healing comes. There was no more denial. Tom was no longer on Earth to enjoy, but alive in Heaven. I longed for a major key in my life and wanted to be finished with the minor key of grief. It felt like a major eclipse occurred and there was a hole in my heart and soul. Even though I knew God does all things well, I continued to ask Him questions but reminded myself that I needed to trust Him.

What I did know was God had a purpose and He does not owe me an explanation of His plan. However, I felt thankful for the opportunity God gave us to offer life for others through organ donation, which I considered a gift. I tried to tell my sadness to go away, but it would not. It took a bit of energy to smile and maintain it even though I tried. Friends validated that God was going to use me to promote organ donation and help others through their grief, which was encouraging. But I was not ready yet.

One of the requirements for the Gender Issues class was to choose a gender issue topic, work together as a group, consisting of another female and male, and create a presentation regarding gender issues. I suggested grief and gender issues, and my partners agreed. I wrote a play about a married couple whose adolescent son committed suicide. We analyzed how males and females respond during grief as we acted out the scenario. It helped to enhance my healing and educated the class. When we finished, several members of the class commented, 'So how do we top this presentation?'

I then further illustrated the "Stepping Stones," by Barbara Williams, a poem regarding the process of grief. I cut out paper bags in the shape of stepping stones and labeled them with shock, denial, anger, loneliness, grief, despair, and finally, acceptance—somewhat shadowing the five stages brought forth by Elisabeth Kubler-Ross. I laid the paper stones on the floor and took the hand of a classmate to illustrate how we need others to help us through this process until we can do it alone. Once enough healing occurs, the poet feels we are ready to help others through this process. It felt profound and encouraging.

Whenever I had the opportunity in my classes, I educated others on organ donation. I included it in my research class and shared my story in classes professors requested, such as in Health and Mental Health and loss and grief. Sharing Tom's story propelled me to educate the public on organ donation and contributed to my healing.

I found grief pulverizes you and leads to a clearer sense of priorities, heightened empathy, and intimacy. I now found myself saying, 'I love you,' when completing a face-to-face encounter or ending a phone conversation with a close friend or family member. I also sensed a heightened sense of fear and vulnerability. Among them was losing another son, my only child left, as well as facing my own mortality."

Further Correspondence from the Heart Recipient

One source of comfort for Janet became her increasing contact with the recently identified recipient of Tom's heart. As the fall of 1998 got underway within the town of Niagara Falls, the confluence of messages traveling between herself, Pete, and other members of the Radigan family would form an inevitable path toward a physical meeting. As she recalled in an October 1998 journal entry:

"At the end of October, I received a letter from the public education manager from UNYTS, stating she received a letter from the heart recipient, as well as from his sister. She apologized again as to the reason there was a delay in forwarding the correspondence from Columbia.

These letters were written on September 6th and 7th, and UNYTS had just recently received them in October. The coordinator from Columbia Hospital indicated that she sent them 'To Whom It May Concern.' The public education manager provided the coordinator her direct name, address, and phone number so they would be sent directly to her at UNYTS. She also encouraged me to communicate directly to the heart recipient when I felt comfortable doing so. I felt somewhat frustrated receiving these letters through the UNYTS, the Organ Procurement Organization (OPO), which takes time.

Reading these letters was wonderful, heartwarming, and surreal. Each letter brought more confidence about my desire to meet the heart recipient. He shared a lot of Tom's characteristics, mirroring his, which felt pleasant, interesting to hear, and comforting. I always knew I wanted to meet the heart recipient if he was willing since the heart is the emotional center of the soul. I felt open to meeting other recipients, as well, but wanted to meet the heart recipient first.

His sister's letter expressed her intense gratitude that her brother was alive due to organ donation, expressing her deep love for her brother and everything he endured. As with other families, donation changed their lives, as well. She encouraged me to meet their family in the future. I could not read these letters without sadness, tears, and gratitude since I was offered that privilege. I shared them with Tim, friends, and family, who were moved with the gratitude they expressed."

Letter from Pete's Sister (Tracey)

September 6, 1998

Dear Jan,

A few minutes ago, I got off the phone with my mother. She read the letter you wrote to my brother. After I hung up with my mother I was in tears. For you, because of your loss and making probably one of the most difficult decisions you ever had to make. And for our family, because your son gave my brother the gift of life. The way you described Tom is exactly how my brother is. He is a young vibrant man who has always put others before himself. He is my only brother, and I do not know what my life would be like without him in it. Every day I thank God for the gift your son gave my brother. Your son lives on in my brother and his positive energy and views on life make my brother the luckiest man alive. I believe my brother was left on this earth to tell and show others how precious life is and how people take advantage of the life God has given them. He has always had a positive attitude and appreciated the small things in life that others took for granted. Now, that outlook on life has so much more meaning, thanks to Tom. You have no idea how your son, Tom, and your decision to donate his organs, has changed our family and our attitude towards life itself. I had to write this letter to you because you have changed my life forever. I love my brother and Tom because now they are one. Your son is now my brother, too. They are a perfect match. I hope we will have the chance in the future to meet so our family can thank you in person.

Sincerely,

Tracey Radigan-Sabino

Letter from Pete

September 7, 1998

Dear Jan,

I received your most welcome letter from the hospital this past Thursday, September 3, 1998. Ironically, I was with another donor family, speaking with the president of the National Coalition on Donation in Philadelphia, PA. A good friend of mine was next to me when I got the message off my answering machine at work. He is also a heart recipient. I grabbed his arm and out loud I proclaimed you had written me.

Going through the ordeal that was my heart transplant was traumatic and it was difficult at times for me and my family. However, nothing compares to the ordeal that you and your family went through and will continue to go through. I am happy that you found solace in my first letter. I am not sure where the letter got held up, but it does not matter. What matters is that you received it.

Your son, Tom, was a special person. When my mother, father, and four sisters read your letter it brought them to tears. You see, your son's personality mirrors my own based on your description. I am very energetic, outgoing, and have been described as having a keen ability to look at events in the scheme of a broad-based picture. Ask the OPO for the letters by at least one of my sisters. My mother is trying to put her thoughts into words.

My friend thinks that he saw you at the reception in Ohio placing a swatch of a motorcycle on the national quilt. He believes he took a picture. It is a small world. I am not sure if I mentioned it to you in my last letter, but two donor families, three heart recipients, and myself formed a non-profit organization called Transplant Speakers International (TSI). I have seen too much life and death around transplantation for me not to use the gift of life your son gave to me to help others lead fuller lives with less pain. I say this in my prayers every morning and night.

It was ironic that you talked about the Kidney Foundation meeting for donor families and transplant recipient families being held in Philadelphia, PA in October. Most of my family will be there along with some other members of the TSI board. If you are able, and you would like to meet, please contact your Organ Procurement Organization (OPO) and ask them to contact my hospital, and the coordinator will contact me, and we can arrange a meeting. Though I would love to meet you and thank you in person, I understand if this would be too difficult, and I will continue correspondence in this fashion.

Thank you for your kind words and I too hope that my words provide some continued comfort amidst your loss. I hope and anticipate continued correspondence as well.

Pete

Tom's Heart Recipient

For Janet, the two letters would serve as a boosting source of strength and the force which would demolish the final barrier toward meeting the Radigans. After weeks of thought and reflection, on December 12, 1998, she submitted three letters acknowledging her new intention. The first went to Pete's sister, Tracey, the second to Pete, and a third to the public education manager at UNYTS.

Letter to Tracey

December 12, 1998

Dear Tracey,

Thank you for your most kind and thoughtful words regarding Tom and your brother's heart transplant. I was emotionally touched through your expression of sympathy and your gratitude of life regarding your brother Pete, and how it has strongly influenced you and your family. Their similar qualities are most amazing. I am appreciative your brother uses his gift of life to impact the lives of others.

Weeks after the funeral, several people questioned my ex-husband and myself regarding how we made the decision to donate Tom's organs, stating their reluctance to donate if presented with the decision. I feel compelled to tell you the story so you might know.

On a warm summer night of August 2, 1997, about 11:15 pm, I just finished a conversation with a friend of mine on the telephone. As I headed to my bedroom to prepare for bed, the telephone rang, and my ex-husband informed me of our son's motorcycle accident and that he was being transported via mercy-flight to the trauma center in Western New York.

Tom had lived with his father in the country for almost four years. His father found him lying in the road about two miles from his home shortly after the accident and saw movement in Tom's extremities. Hearing this, being a nurse, I prepared in my mind that perhaps the accident was not life-threatening but serious and thus I prayed. Later, we learned that after he was ejected from the motorcycle, he hit her windshield, causing a severe cerebral injury and then unconsciousness. He then flew 178 feet backward before landing on the road, with the motorcycle being dragged another 252 feet before stopping.

As the medical staff assessed him, I waited in the emergency waiting room. At 2 AM, the neurosurgeon called us in to inform us about Tom's condition. Being as tactful and kind as he could be, he explained that the trauma caused extensive bleeding and swelling which eventually leads to brainstem compression and herniation, which is always fatal.

He stated that we had two choices, "Either to support him until he dies or do surgery to relieve the intracranial pressure and remove severely injured brain tissue." He presented the grave picture that even though there would be a five percent chance of recovery with surgery, Tom would never talk again, and at best remain in a vegetative state. After hearing those words, I said, "Lord, please take him quickly." It was like a knife being thrust into my heart—a parent's worst nightmare!! In concluding his conversation with us, he said, "You may want to consider organ donation."

After the neurosurgeon left the room, I looked at Tom's father and said, "I only know of one thing to do and that is to pray—do you mind if I pray?" He said, "No." I proceeded to pray after taking his hand and thanked God for lending Tom to us for almost 17 years and then asked for His wisdom and strength for what was ahead. Tom's father returned to the outside of the emergency room where he had previously been waiting with the parents of the girl who hit him. Their first question to him was how is Tom? He said, "They are waiting for him to die!" It was an agonizing moment for all involved.

Although Tom remained unresponsive and his breathing aided by a respirator, we talked to him, hugged him, and assured him of our love. We both knew beyond a shadow of a doubt that organ transplant would be imperative. Being a nurse, I knew the medical diseases that destroy and debilitate people, and we both knew that Tom, being a giving person, would want to share his life with others. Understanding that death meant separation of the body from the spirit and that at death Tom's spirit would be in Heaven, we knew he would no longer need his body. We notified the neurosurgeon that organ donation was our choice if Tom did not survive.

Knowing as parents we needed to attempt any minuscule chances for survival, we opted for surgery which began at approximately 4 AM on August 3rd. Post-operatively, the surgeon informed us that the trauma was worse than expected. Spontaneous breathing, although supported by a respirator, was the only factor preventing the neurosurgeon from pronouncing him clinically dead in surgery. Breathing tests were performed every six hours or so, and as soon as spontaneous breathing deteriorated due to gradual brainstem compression, he would be pronounced dead.

When my other son arrived at the hospital from Savannah, Georgia, he asked the neurosurgeon if there was anything that could be done, and he said, "There's nothing else we can do, he's in God's hands." Each breathing test evidenced continued deterioration until finally on August 4th at 4:03 PM, he was pronounced dead.

I hugged my precious son, told him that I LOVED him for the very last time, that I would MISS him tremendously, and that he was now SAFE in his Heavenly Father's Arms. Walking away, I said goodnight, because I know I will see him again someday!

My comfort comes from knowing Tom saved four lives (including Pete's), helped many others through organ transplants and bone and tissue donation. Tom suffered no pain. The accident was not his fault, nor did he injure anyone. My prayers were answered in that he was taken quickly, and he is experiencing eternal life in Heaven. Even though it is indeed an earthly tragedy, I consider it a heavenly mercy due to the circumstances, and thus I am at peace with his death. The miracle of no injuries below his head after being thrown 178 feet further confirms to me as stated in my letter to Pete, that God perfectly plans having people like your brother in His Plan. He assured me that I am profoundly grateful that your brother Pete was chosen to have a second chance at life!

I indicated in Pete's letter that I gave my OPO permission to give him my name, address, and telephone number so we can correspond directly. I anticipate meeting you all in person when we can arrange it and sharing your difficulties and experiences relative to the transplant. I think meeting with you will help tremendously in my own personal healing. Your sympathy and gratitude have been much appreciated. Thank you again for taking the time to write and have a Merry Christmas!

Jan, my precious son's mother

Letter to Pete

December 12, 1998

Dear Pete,

I became overcome with heartfelt emotion as I read your letter of September 7, 1998. Your sister's letter thrilled my heart as well, and I have enclosed a letter to her. If I could sum up the feelings regarding Tom's loss and your gift of life, I would not have guessed that such intense feelings of sorrow and joy could co-exist. Veteran grievers warned me the second year would be harder, and indeed I find it so. His absence saddens me, especially with the holiday season coming upon us. Because Tom loved Christmas, his spirit will be profoundly missed as past Christmas memories reflect his life, love, and giving. Fortunately, his brother plans on coming home for Christmas, which will help ease the loss.

I am reminded, however, that through Christ's birth and death, we who have accepted His gift of salvation experience life. Tom, through his death, gave his ALL so others could live. Even though I felt sad, I found consolation that four lives were given a second chance (including yours), and others were enhanced. Absence of internal injuries, after being thrown 178 feet from the impact, confirms to me that God perfectly plans, because otherwise transplant would have been impossible. I am confident that God does ALL things well, even though it hurts tremendously, and I do not understand.

I received your letter a few days after the National Kidney Foundation Conference in Philadelphia. As you probably deduced, I was unable to attend due to unexpected responsibilities. Regarding the reception in Ohio last August, I did place a swatch on the national quilt, but it was not a motorcycle. I would be happy to share these memories through pictures when we meet.

I am ecstatic that you are able to impact the lives of others through speaking and forming TSI. I look forward to hearing more about it. Tom is cheering you all the way because he would have done the same! Thank you for sharing how similar your personality is to Tom's. I trust your body continues to accept Tom's heart. I have given my OPO permission to give you my address for future contact, knowing that direct correspondence will be much more efficient. I look forward to meeting you and your family in the future. By the way, have you had any cravings for hot peppers? Tom loved them as well as salsa and taco chips!!!

Have a Merry Christmas as you continue to celebrate your life.

Jan, "your donor's mom"

Letter Going to the Public Educator at UNYTS

Dear Delia:

Thank you so much for your efforts regarding efficient forwarding of correspondence between myself, the donor family, and the heart recipient from New York whose name is Pete.

Enclosed you will find three copies of letters for the heart recipient Pete and his sister. Pete has conveyed in the past letter his desire to correspond directly, and I agree with him. You have my permission to give him my name, address, and telephone number. I know this is short notice, but I did not know if it might be possible to fax these letters to Columbia so they might arrive before Christmas. Could you also check to see if Pete received a picture of Tom that I sent to him in August? At that time, you stated that Columbia did not feel he was ready to see it.

As previously noted, would you contact me via phone when you receive this letter and when he receives it? I appreciate it very much. Perhaps from that point on, we can directly correspond. Thank you again for your help and have a Merry Christmas.

Sincerely,

Janet Mauk

11

Closer to Meeting

With the forces of two-way communication now in motion, a meeting became inevitable. Pete's power of persuasion, which had helped him greatly in his sales life, was now combined with the Radigans' desire to meet the woman responsible for making the decision that saved the life of their son and brother.
Along with Jan's newfound desire to reach out and meet the family, a confluence of events would quickly lead to a personal "Thank You."
The letters continued during the final month of 1998, as chronicled by Jan in her journal.

December 20, 1998

"The florist came to the door to deliver a Christmas poinsettia from the heart recipient. It was beautiful, and I broke down and cried. I felt thankful for his thoughtfulness and enjoyed the beautiful poinsettia. I missed Tom a lot, but I'm thankful that Pete described himself like Tom in many ways.

The card said, "Dear Jan and family, Have a healthy and happy holiday. I look forward to seeing you soon."

He left his phone number and address. I was still excited but feeling cautious.

WOW! That was a relief. Now we could correspond directly whenever we chose."

December 22, 1998

"I was out for the evening and when I returned there was a message on my answering machine from Pete. He called and said he knew what to say but was at a loss for words when he left a message. He left his phone number and asked me to call him if I wanted to. So at 9:30 p.m. that night, feeling nervous and excited at the same time, I called him.

We talked for two hours. It was incredible! I thanked him for the poinsettia he sent. It was hard to imagine. WOW!!! I was talking to the man who had Tom's heart!! I felt like I had a kinship with him. I cannot explain. I feel like he is a friend, a 'son,' and a brother. We exchanged email addresses and shared the many miracles we both experienced. It was a breath of fresh air and a wonderful experience. I felt ecstatic and could hardly fall asleep! He later stated his only regret was that he had to get off the telephone. Pete told me of his plans to travel to Toronto for work in early February and he would like to meet me.

He went on to share how he had developed a virus at 21 which attacked his heart when he was a senior in college. He developed hypertrophic myocardial myopathy. He did not know he had it until he had developed congestive heart failure while presenting at a sales meeting. It took him a long time to walk to his car, and he knew something was wrong. He said, 'I am 33, athletic, six feet tall, big-boned, and my little sister, who lives with me, says that I am sexy (laugh).' Pete had completed his Masters Degree in Business in November of 1997 after receiving the heart transplant. He traveled as a sales trainer for Ricoh.

Pete also said he knew the lung recipients, and they were doing well. I asked him how he knew them. As it turned out, Pete, his family, and the prospective lung recipients and their families all met in the surgical unit before their transplants. The doctor stated these three organs came from the same donor.

Pete was in the hospital from April to August, when Tom died. He said his hospital room overlooked the Hudson River, and he watched jet skiers on the water while wishing someone would die so he could live. He said his mother feels guilty because she prayed every day he would live.

I read the letter I received from UNYTS to him. Pete corrected it, saying he was not engaged. I inquired whether he received Tom's picture; and he said no, they would not give it to him. They said the only way they would give it to him would be if I flew to New York City, and we both took psychological tests. He said they were not going to give me your home address, but someone on the Q-T' did. He asked me if I would be interested in speaking, writing, and teaching. He found when donor families and recipients spoke together, it made a phenomenal impact. I felt excited!!!"

December 24, 1998

"My son, Tim, called stating he had received his Christmas presents from me and he would call me tomorrow. He told me he may have to go to Korea. I spent time with friends on Christmas Eve."

December 25, 1998 (Christmas Day)

"I received a book on grief at Christmas from a friend. One of the passages stated, 'The reason we feel so deeply is due to our capacity to love and dedicate our emotions and energies to others. It is these that cause our pain as they come rushing in the void left from your loved one.' This further normalized my feelings and thoughts. I was in no mood to face another Christmas; and every time I thought about Christmas, I would cry, missing Tom.

I went through the motions of Christmas, but my heart was not there. Even though I spent Christmas with loving friends, no one could fill the void of missing Tom. Tim called as he unwrapped his presents. He felt thankful for the presents and disappointed he could not come home. I traveled to the cemetery and left a small balloon and rose at Tom's gravesite, feeling sad and missing Tom. The bitter wind and temperatures made it challenging to stay long. So I came home and wrote my feelings in a poem.

Soon after, Pete called to wish me a MERRY CHRISTMAS, which was the BEST Christmas present I received, as it distracted me from my intense sadness.

Pete asked me two questions. 'Would I be willing to speak with him on organ donation, and would I be interested in co-authoring a book with him?' He said he did not think there was any published book written by the donor family and the recipient together. Immediately, I said 'YES!' It was another miracle and direction in the middle of my steadfast grief.

Pete said his family was apprehensive about talking with me, but after his dad began the conversation and broke the ice, everyone relaxed. His dad told me his son was phenomenal, stating I would agree when I meet him. He further explained Pete felt passionate about educating the public about organ donation, already touching many lives. He wanted his life to count.

I talked with everyone in the family, and they expressed their love and gratitude for Tom's heart and Pete's second chance at life. It helped to bring a connection to Tom and COMFORT ME on a most difficult day. Each person talked with me and inquired how I was doing since they knew it would be an emotional encounter.

Pete showed sensitivity and caring, giving me permission to stop conversing anytime if I became overwhelmed emotionally. His mom spoke to me, expressing her sympathy over Tom's death, and commented on the beautiful letters I wrote. She said they all prayed before Pete's surgery. His oldest sister, Kerry, spoke with me next. She has three children and delivered a son, Brennan Peter, during Pete's stay in the hospital. She relayed that Brennan was on life support, almost died, but improved. She said she had a small idea of what I must have gone through.

Kerry went on to say that every time Pete speaks, he ends his talk with the poem "To Remember Me," (printed in the back of this book) as they cry together. His other sister, Tracey, has two children, two years old, and six months. Jeanie, his youngest sister, was pregnant and told me how much she appreciated the letter I sent her. She said, 'I am always here for you, Jan.' Pete's sisters all commented that he was a great brother, and his heart transplant changed their lives.

These captivating moments of love and gratitude abounded, as my ambivalent feelings of loss and gratitude coexisted. Speaking with Pete and his family was the only gift that held any meaning and the best Christmas present I received. Words cannot explain the impact of their love and gratitude as they helped to bring a connection to Tom and comfort to me on a most difficult day. It was a bright light during the darkness of grief. Friends and family were excited, as well, as I shared the phone conversations with them. My mood lifted some, as I also felt excited about my new direction of speaking, educating, supporting, and writing. Contact with Pete seemed to open doors in multiple areas, and he networked well."

December 28, 1998

"Pete thanked me through an email for speaking with his family on Christmas, writing that it was uplifting and filled a void in his life."

The void both Pete and Janet shared through their transplant experience would be closed quickly. The email exchanges grew in frequency and length, and for the final days of 1998 and opening weeks of 1999, updates of 500-1,000 words were becoming the norm. Jan wrote about her return

to school while Pete conveyed his feelings about returning to work.
Sometimes, the tone was light.

Although their words were shared, they still seemed to be arriving at each
other from complex shadows within the AOL and Outlook mail servers.
Pete and Janet were virtual allies but could bump into each other on the
street and be unaware of the significance of the chance encounter. They still
had no idea what the other looked like, as recapped by Janet in her journal
during the first week of 1999.

January 5, 1999

"Pete sent me an email and he received Tom's pictures, saying it took
him three hours to open the envelope. He is sending me a picture of
him and his family, as well."

January 6, 1999

"I received pictures of Pete and his family. It was nice to put faces to
names. I also contacted Delia from UNYTS and informed her Pete
and I would be meeting in the future. I also signed up for the
UNYTS volunteer orientation later in the month. I felt ready to start
giving back. She encouraged me, stating it would be great if Pete and
I could speak together. I shared the impact he had in speaking to
many people in the past year and his formation of Transplant
Speakers International (TSI). She stated that she would plan on
obtaining media attention if we did speak separately or together."

January 7, 1999

"I kept thinking of Pete in his picture and I stared at his chest trying
to imagine Tom's heart inside. It is unimaginable. I knew it was
surgically possible, but WOW! To give life to someone else, what a
gift. I felt grateful, we said YES to donation.

We started planning on my visit to New Jersey in March where I would also meet the lung recipient, Joe, and participate in media events and attend a support meeting that Pete and his family attended. It felt exciting to think about and to also know we planned on meeting each other in Toronto on February 4, 1999, exactly one and a half years following Tom's death."

In the final month before their meeting, the emails were transmitted on an almost daily basis. As soon as one person had news to share, the other would quickly receive it. Janet, who had already spoken with Pete and his family, was now free to send pictures, tell family stories, and bond with Pete, who was walking, talking, and breathing because of the heart she had carried inside of her for nine months.

Some missives were chock full of small talk, but Pete enjoyed telling Janet about the work being done with the Transplant Speakers, which was raising hundreds of thousands of dollars while conducting numerous fundraisers across America. In one instance, members of the New York Giants and Jets played a game of pickup football at Fairleigh Dickinson University, with the financial goal set at $100,000. Several of Pete's doctors from Columbia Presbyterian were urged to support the cause with financial help or by spreading the word.

One of the group's cardiologists from the hospital, Dr. Mehmet Oz, already becoming better known for his syndicated television show, transferred $10,000 from his own foundation to TSI.

By the middle of January 1999, a face-to-face meeting was imminent. Pete's job was about to take him to Toronto and in a location close enough to visit Janet in Niagara Falls. But the timing was not right, or so it appeared. The Army was about to ship her son, Tim Mauk, to Korea; and she planned to travel to Savannah to see him before his departure, which was the same weekend she and Pete planned to meet in Toronto. But fate had another plan, and so did the Army. On January 10th, Janet composed an elongated email for her newest friend, and the paragraph in the middle set the wheels in motion for a personal meeting in Toronto.

Janet Wrote to Pete

"On a lighter note, I've decided not to visit my son in Savannah at the beginning of February. Even though he received orders for Korea, he does not believe he will go because of his pending discharge next November. As a result of that decision, would you reconsider meeting each other while you are in Toronto at the beginning of next month, as you spoke of before? You can drive down if you like. I would feel more comfortable meeting before our March 11th meeting in New Jersey, if that is possible.

I talked to the public educator from UNYTS the Buffalo OPO regarding our correspondence. She said she was not sure if the New York City transplant services planned to give him my address. So, I explained to her what happened. I told her about TSI and promoting organ donation through his speaking. She said if you two meet it will be the first time (for donor family and recipient to meet) in the history of Buffalo. I expressed great surprise—I could not believe it!! I guess I would not think of not pursuing it. She said after you do meet and at an appropriate time, we will bring in the media!!! Perhaps as time goes on, we will get involved.

I must admit I felt moved at seeing a picture of you and imagining Tom's heart in your chest. It just brought tears to my eyes as I stared at your chest for the longest time trying to comprehend it all as I felt overwhelmed with gratitude. I again felt overjoyed that Tom's death was not a senseless tragedy but had a purpose, one of which was saving the lives of others. It really adds to the healing process. I am so glad you continue to do well. It is a miracle. If I had to choose a potential heart recipient, I could not have chosen better! I am not disappointed at all! I feel doubly blessed. Not only do you have Tom's heart, but you are actively promoting organ donation. God never stops pouring out his blessings during this tragedy. Thanks for allowing me to share my feelings."

Two days later, Janet would write back and apologize for comments about staring at Pete's chest, which was met with a laugh and rebuttal. "Thanks for the concern. I probably would be staring at my chest as well if I were in your shoes."

The final logistical details of the meeting were taking form, and Pete detailed the plans in a January 20ᵗʰ message:

Jan,

I am sitting here in California about to write an email to Columbia Presbyterian Hospital to ask the doctors we have come to know so well to support our next charity event for fundraising for TSI. If I did not mention it to you, it will be some time at the end of March at Fairleigh Dickinson University in Bergen County, New Jersey. It will be a New York Giants vs. New York Jets football game with all the proceeds going to TSI. We hope to raise over $100,000. Our last one was right before Christmas. It was an autograph signing with several players from the New Jersey Devils hockey team, in which we raised $6,324. Not bad for two hours, huh?

Once we get enough money, we can really make TSI fly with wings of its own. I believe this is one of the reasons I was left here on Earth, to use my abilities to help others suffering through the types of things we went through. This does not include only recipients, but also, whenever possible, donor families.

My friend Ed Masol (Board member of TSI with me) also received his heart from the Buffalo OPO. He had not received word in two years. I suggested he contact Delia directly. When he did, he found out she had not received his letters from the hospital. This is a crying shame! I have met hundreds of donor families, some of which are angry the recipient could not even say thank you. However, almost every heart recipient that I know has written a thank you letter. I have traced the problems in New York down to the hospital. Ed was just told, via a letter from Delia, his donor family received his letter and had requested information on how to write to recipients. I cannot tell you how happy I felt for him and for his donor family. I believe there are others who would find solace like we have if contact were made possible, if both parties consented.

Another member of TSI and myself have started a campaign at Columbia to initiate policy reform on this very issue. I offered to set up a roundtable to discuss the issues and update these policies. I look forward to seeing your pictures when I get back. Unfortunately, I get back on Friday and head back to Florida on Sunday. By the way, this is not normal. I usually travel about once a month. This is just a fluke.

These conversations were fortuitous because following their meeting in Toronto, they would schedule a community meeting and for the first time speak together. This was the beginning of what would become the best way to educate the public on organ and tissue donation…from the tragedy of a donor family to the gift of life from the recipients' perspectives.

I am arriving in Toronto on Sunday, January 31, 1999. I would really like to meet you, but it will be difficult if it is two-plus hours to drive to your home and back. Do you have any family near Toronto or friends you would have reason to visit and maybe stay with overnight? Just a thought. If not, I will see how the week goes. Do not worry about overwhelming me. I am not sure how emotional I will be when I see you in person, but I think it will be a great beginning for us.

Wow! I just realized how long I have been rambling in his letter. I am going to try and give you a phone call either tomorrow night or Saturday during the day. Hopefully, we can catch up then.

Talk to you soon, Pete

The final logistical details were hammered out over a dozen more email exchanges, and then the last words as cyber acquaintances were delivered in a pair of emails from Janet on February 2, 1999, the day after her birthday. The tension and excitement were rising.

. . .

February 1, 1999 (12:07 a.m.)

Pete,

I woke up this morning thankful God has granted me another year of life, a year older, or should I say younger, and that I want to impact the lives of others. Yes, it is my birthday!

Since I have not touched the homework today, I must get some sleep and finish it tomorrow. Have a great day tomorrow and I will see you soon!!!

Jan

And for the parting thought –

February 2, 1999 (10:34 p.m.)

Pete,

I hope you are doing fine as we anticipate Thursday. Are you getting more anxious, excited, etc.? I am! Plans seem to be working out on this end. Do you want to meet me in the lobby, do you want me to knock at your door or "play it by ear?" I continue to share my excitement. My friend, Kathy, plans to travel with me. She is one of the most compassionate people I know, is easy to talk with, and fun to be with, and shall I say, Irish??? Remember, if this is too much, let me know. I hope you are enjoying Toronto and had a good day!!! I will see ya soon! - Jan

12

Once in a Lifetime Meeting

(Janet prepares to meet with Pete at last.)

My friend, Kathy and I planned to travel to Toronto and meet Pete on February 4, 1999, exactly 1½ years since Tom's death. We reached the hotel about 5:15 p.m. I felt excited and anxious at the same time, so I asked Kathy to drive my car. Due to my euphoric state, I could have caused a car accident.

Janet and Kathy arrived in Toronto and entered the Westin Prince hotel full of nervous anticipation. For Janet, the feeling was surreal. Not only would she meet the beneficiary of her son's heart but she would also be an arm's length away from the rhythmic memory of Tom. This would be the closest she had been to her son since he passed away one and a half years to the date before. Only this time, his heart would be beating.
In her words...

Meeting the Heart Recipient - Feb. 4, 1999

I wanted to meet him alone and become acquainted and comfortable without the pressures of others around, other than Kathy. I must admit, I felt fearful to share certain things with him because I did not want to overwhelm him with my sadness and perhaps scare him away since survivors' guilt is common with transplant recipients.

I felt comfortable about meeting him and thankful I had a picture of him, However, I felt unsure of what my response would be emotionally. We then signed into room 803.

As we walked into the room, a bouquet of flowers lay on the bed. I felt moved with tears. The card attached to it said, "I thought this card was perfect...just because. Looking forward to seeing you and Kathy." The message on the hotel stationery said, "Please ring my room when you arrive—room 1110."

Initially, his line was busy. I felt happy I brought Kathy with me because I could not function well due to my state of euphoria at meeting him. We finally did reach him, and after some discussion, he decided to come to our room. Kathy had already arranged the flowers in a vase in the room, and I told her she would have to answer the door.

KNOCK, KNOCK!

There was a hallway and a wall as you walked into the room, so Pete could not see me as he walked in. As he turned the corner, I walked toward him and hugged him.

How do you comprehend that Tom's heart is in someone else??? HOW could that be?

I was hoping I would cry but felt more in shock meeting him and trying to believe it all. Just to think, the three letters Y-E-S to donation gave him a chance to live. I just wanted to make sure it was real!! It was unbelievable. We all made ourselves comfortable as he shared his story. Just to think, as he spoke, the doctor tells you that you are going to die if a heart is not found for you? Imagine that? He shared he had made up his last will and testament while he waited for a heart. His family almost lost him twice.

Pete continued to share after the heart transplant that he popped a stitch and bled internally, and was taken back to surgery to control the bleeding. Later, as well, he developed fluid around his heart which caused arrhythmias, and a thoracentesis was performed to remove the fluid.

While in ICU, he experienced psychosis due to the combination of narcotics, anesthetics, and being in ICU for a lengthy stay. He cried, thinking he was losing his mind. He thought the hospital staff was killing his family.

After he went to the step-down unit, he felt fearful of taking any pain medications because of this incident. He improved and hoped to be discharged home, but now he could not stand up, so he spent another few weeks in physical therapy. He had been hospitalized since April 16, 1997, but was hoping to return to his previous job in November. What a miracle that he was alive after all of that.

Pete made reservations at a Japanese restaurant. As we arrived, a group of people who were sitting at a distant table stared at us as we walked in. Pete told me they were the group he trained that day, and he had shared with them about the meeting. He said, "Jan, if you think this is hard to believe for you and me, it is even harder for others." He introduced me to the group, who were awe-stricken. Two women in front had tears in their eyes.

We then enjoyed a five-course meal where the chef prepared the food in front of us. I was glad Kathy was with me due to the intensity of the situation. Pete previously stated he could be sarcastic and direct, and with their Irish heritage, they teased one another, which brought some welcomed laughter and levity to the situation.

After a couple of hours, Pete suggested we return to our room so I could share the story of Tom's death. Before we left, we noticed the group he had taught leaving the room. One salesman stopped and talked to us, moved by our story, stating we were an inspiration to him. He said that if we had not made our decision to say yes to donation, Pete would not be here.

We left the restaurant and walked through the halls to the lobby where we took pictures together. We proceeded to the room and made ourselves comfortable. I started Tom's story at birth, sharing his struggles with ADHD, school, sharing the last three years of his life. I told him I knew something bad was going to happen to Tom and how God prepared me.

I took him through the hospital experience, the viewing, funeral, and burial. At one point, I started to cry. Pete took my hand and said he has a part of Tom. He gave me permission to complete the story another time if I chose. I felt very scattered and asked Kathy several times what was next, or did I forget anything? She was helpful and told me she did not know how I did it. She had direct eye contact with Pete and saw tears well up in his eyes several times.

When I finally finished the story, Pete wanted to know if we wanted to see his surgical scar, which I was not expecting. He opened his shirt to show us. It was reality. Not that I did not believe it, but it was unfathomable. The most poignant moment occurred when he asked me if I wanted to listen to my son's heart, now his.

I put my head on his chest and listened. It was not like listening to the quality, rhythm, or rate of a heartbeat or detecting arrhythmias, which I practiced as a nurse. Listening to his heart brought a connection to Tom, joy to my soul, in contrast to the previous sadness, as tears formed in my eyes. I felt choked up listening, trying to imagine the entire situation. The sound of his heartbeat was a melody to my ear, as I wanted to permanently affix my head to his chest to hear it continually. It brought comfort to me.

Pete departed shortly after to talk with his family. Neither one of us slept much that night due to our excitement. Kathy helped me process the events of the evening.

The next morning, we met, and I listened to his heart again, not wanting to leave. To think Tom's heart had beat within my body for nine months and was now in him, was incredible. I started tearing up again, and we hugged as we both became emotional.

As we signed out, the desk clerk asked how I liked the flowers, which Kathy had. The clerk stated she had placed them in the room, and they thought it was a secret admirer. We said no, asking if they knew anything about it. Of course, they did not. As we proceeded to tell them, they were astonished as well.

After I dropped Kathy off in Buffalo, I began processing everything I experienced as I traveled to my home. Melodies danced in my head with the feeling of overwhelming gratitude, as the minor key of grief began to change to a major key. When I returned home, I penned this poem.

. . .

MELODY OF LOVE

Meeting you and hearing the beating of your heart
brings melodies to my soul
I could never imagine.

As streams of tears well up in my eyes
I'm reminded of songs in a minor key
that have played in my heart in recent bygone days.

Songs of shock, denial, disbelief, and sadness
emanated from my heart like staccato notes.

Struggling to find a major key seemed unreachable
as the process of grief prevented a key change.

Keenly listening to your heartbeat, the beautiful harmony
Blended smoothly as it reflected love, joy, purpose, and hope.
It was the playing of those notes I long for and never tire of.

The time is now where the melody in a major key
or the joy of your chance at life helps diminish,
the minor key or the grief of the loss of my son.

Thank you for sharing your heart, as its rhythm and notes
combine to complete the melody that
will play on in my soul forever.

Each heartbeat reminds me of melodies of love for Tom,
as memories of him will forever be indelibly etched in my heart.
It is the void of his loss linked with your gratitude overflowing,
that helps to heal the emptiness without my son,
and serves a purpose beyond the tragedy itself.

Thank you for helping me change
the key in this melody of love!
Your "donor mom," Jan

I sent this to Pete after I wrote it, feeling full of gratitude.

———————

(Pete expressed his thoughts about Janet's poem.)

"When I received this from Jan, I remember feeling that a poem conveys so many different things. Jan's poem took me on a journey of love and compassion I will not soon forget. I paused often to collect my emotions as I attempted to understand the tragedy she and her family endured. And yet, she celebrated the gift of life with me by saying yes."

13

Moving Forward

Pete always taught that until the public can put a name…a face…and a personality with organ donation and transplantation that it would not be real. It would just be a statistic. From the moment Jan and Pete first spoke, it was like lightning! For the first time, the mother of an organ donor and her heart recipient spoke with raw emotion about the tragedy and death of a loved one that allowed a family in the worst moment of their life to provide the gift of life. First, there was Jan telling her story raw and firsthand with emotion. It was powerful! Then as if Jan bringing tears to everyone's eyes was not enough, Pete shares his story and the triumph he felt by receiving the gift of life through Tom's heart. Here was a woman whose son's heart was beating in the chest of a man she was speaking with side by side. How can organ and tissue donation education ever be the same?

Janet continued her journey.

I completed my volunteer training at UNYTS in January 1999 a few weeks before meeting with Pete. At that point, media opportunities exploded. Whenever UNYTS needed a speaker, they would contact me to check my availability. Until I met Pete, and in the few times

UNYTS asked me to speak, I talked only from my perspective as a donor mother.

In March, I traveled to New Jersey where I met Tom's lung recipient, Joe. Pete, Joe, and I were interviewed by the media and featured in newspapers. I visited Columbia Presbyterian Hospital, where Pete resided for four months while waiting for a heart. I walked through the foyer where the lifesaving organs came through to save the lives of three people—Pete, Joe, and John. Through this hallway, in a profound way, I entered into the lives of Tom's organ recipients. I felt relief to be walking out of my room of grief for a time and into their lives, attempting to feel their pain and struggles. Pete also introduced me to medical personnel who cared for him. I could only imagine how challenging it would be to wait and wonder and if an organ would become available. Profound because this was part of the journey Tom took to save lives.

When possible, we would try to speak together, which included Nurses Education Day at Erie County Medical Center in Buffalo, New York, and the annual Nurses Education Day in Western New York. On April 8th, we spoke together at the Salvation Army in Niagara Falls, inviting the public to attend. As one participant would state, "Either of you could be effective speakers alone, but speaking together, sharing your stories, leaves the audience speechless!" In early April 1999,, the local 8-year-old kidney recipient and his family came to my house to meet me and thank me. His mother stated this was the healthiest her son had ever been. He no longer needed dialysis treatments. This warmed my heart, and I knew Tom would smile knowing he helped a child. The next day, the meeting was posted on the bottom of the front page of the *Buffalo News*. The top part reported the deadly shootings at Columbine. One person told me the top of the paper was about senseless deaths and the bottom about restoring life, which was refreshing to observe.

Other speaking engagements included the kidney transplant group, as I spoke about writing to donor families and thanking them for their kidneys. What an incredibly powerful year and a half this was for both Pete and me regarding the conglomeration of events. What I did not know was how this would contribute toward my healing.

I was notified in June of 2000 that UNYTS, now Connect Life, chose me for a community service award which would be presented at a dinner in September of 2000. The pathway to that night culminated through the ongoing process of educating the public on organ donation through Pete and my efforts.

September of 2000 brought the culmination of our speaking efforts together, as Pete and Joe presented me with the Community Service Award. Even though I felt honored, it was more touching that both the heart and lung recipient traveled here to present it to me. There was a standing ovation. It was the culmination of Tom's wish, of saying yes to donation. Tom's heart truly came full circle. I was moved to tears by the tragedy of losing Tom but also by the triumph of seeing the result of saying yes to donation, as his transplant recipients could now enjoy life once more. Now it was easier to see God's plan fulfilled, according to His merciful will. The Gift of Life clearly shows the tragedy and triumph of organ, tissue, and eye donation and its importance through the ongoing process of educating the public through Pete and my efforts. This changed the face of public speaking on organ/tissue/eye donation.

Looking out at the audience after I received the award and expressed my gratitude, I realized educating others on organ donation came alive in front of their eyes, the result of their hard work to save lives. As Pete says, "They can now put names, faces, and personalities with organ donation and the gift of life in transplantation."

While there was delight for Pete Radigan in his newfound life and a growing friendship with Janet, his donor mother, and their new connection on speaking, there presented consequences as he learned to live with his new heart. His job with Ricoh became more challenging as the company requested that he consider less physically demanding options. Because he trained others nationally, in essence, the company hoped he would settle for an office job with no travel.

Post-Transplant Dating Game

Pete's personal life remained difficult, as well. When he first became ill, he had a serious girlfriend; but the stress of facing a future with an ailing husband caused her to have a meltdown of sorts.

Pete recalled, "She became stressed and it stressed out my family because she could not handle the events and uncertainty of the future. As a result, prior to the transplant, I decided to break things off permanently."

The worry over finding true love again engulfed Pete.

"The biggest challenge that remained was how to date. Dating becomes challenging itself, but determining when and how to tell someone about my transplant posed a problem. She could be the most cavalier woman in the world, but she may wonder, *Do I really want to deal with this?* That is what caused me to want to wait to tell someone. However, if I waited, I did not want the person I was going to start to build a relationship with to think I did not trust her enough to tell her immediately. The proverbial 'Catch-22' dilemma."

But Pete's life mission had changed. Enlisting help from fellow transplant survivors Frank Bodino and Ed Masol, the trio sought to educate others about the power of organ donation. Their collective effort resulted in the formation of Transplant Speakers International (TSI). The idea was Pete's, but as Bodino recalled, the final product was the work of many.

"Pete was an ambitious guy," said Bodino. "He was always talking about his idea of a speakers bureau. Eventually, the three of us put together a program and went around the country teaching transplant recipients how to speak about their experiences."

The project was a year in the making and grew to include great input from

Janet, who spoke at many of the events and contributed mightily to the growing media interest, which included exposure at the local and national levels.

Pete's charisma and chutzpah always worked to his advantage, even in his recovery state. Back in New Jersey, he took a solo trip to Paramus Park Mall one day, unaware his verbal skills would change his life once again. Stopping off for a quick lunch before heading back to work for Transplant Speakers International, he looked up from his sandwich and was instantly mesmerized by the sight in front of him. She was Spanish, Colombian perhaps? Maybe Portuguese? In an instant, he decided to find out. Walking to the nearby table, he began the inquiry of the beautiful Spanish woman and her friend.

"Are you girls from Colombia?" This began a mutual dialogue, somewhat serious, somewhat playful, and somewhat rebellious. Pete dropped his business card in front of one of the women, named Giselle.

"I do not want that," she exclaimed.

"Call me," responded Pete. "I'll be kicking myself all night if I leave here without telling you that I want to take you to dinner."

"And then he left," recalled Giselle. "My friend put his card in my handbag, and I went home to Fairview (New Jersey) and forgot all about it." Two days later, she was reminded when his card fell out of her purse.

"It was 9:00 p.m. on a Saturday," said Giselle. "I saw he was a manager at Ricoh. But I was not ready to pick up the phone yet."

It would be another week and a half before she made the decision to call.

"Who's this?" Unfortunately, Pete's memory failed him after ten days. And for a second, he thought his hearing had done the same. "I am having trouble understanding you."

"My English was horrible," admitted Giselle.

Coupled with her rapid-fire delivery, it was difficult to pick up on what she was saying, especially since Pete was vacationing at the family beach house. But their combined efforts led to a four-hour talk lasting until 2:00 a.m., ending with a promise they would go out when Pete returned from his business trip in Chicago. Their first date almost imploded before it could begin. Pete suggested a spot called the Big Red Tomato on Jersey's Route 46 in Ft. Lee, the last exit before Weehawken. As if getting lost on the way to the restaurant was not enough, Giselle had neglected to explain the social mores of her fellow Brazilians.

"If you want to invite someone from Brazil, and want to meet at 6:00, you tell them 4:00. We are always one-two hours late." At the scheduled meeting time, Giselle later admitted to Pete that she was working on her hair. However, she did beat the one-hour lag period, and by her own admission was only 45-50 minutes late. Fortunately, she had remembered to select a perfect outfit.

"I wore a sleek, all-black dress," which made Pete forget she was late. The remainder of the evening went very well. "We had dinner, and I asked him questions," said Giselle. "What do you do, where do you live?" The answers obviously pleased her, as a second date was arranged.

Pete was anxious to see Giselle again. Although he was petrified to tell her about his transplant, he was determined to be honest and upfront. In the past, he gauged when to let a girlfriend know about his transplant. His decision to wait was ill-advised, and the relationship ended poorly. When his girlfriend found out about the transplant, she called the person who had introduced them and was upset that she had not been told the truth from the beginning.
Rather than wait and hope for a happy outcome, he decided to be

proactive. There was a business trip to Chicago coming up, and the decision was made to put everything out in the open and hope for the best.

"Giselle met me at Newark (Airport) after the trip, and we agreed to meet in Hoboken for dinner the following weekend. But I was paranoid about everything." In a sense, so was Giselle. The nightly phone calls were productive, but she was having a hard time believing everything Pete was telling her.

"(Peter) was telling me that he was 34 years old but had no kids, no ex-wife, no child support. I kept thinking to myself—he's lying!"

If Pete had known about the skepticism, he may have delayed the moment of truth. But as they arrived at the restaurant in Hoboken, the time to change his mind had almost completely run out. He ordered wine and they selected their entrees. They then settled down to talk, with the conversation flowing as easily as always. The fact that they both were friendly, outgoing people helped make for a good match. But the length and quality of their future relationship were about to be put to the test. Pete was too anxious to wait until they ate before broaching the topic. He needed to share with her.

"I knew there was only one way to find out if we were going to have a future." With one last inhale, he doubled down on his heart and started speaking. "Giselle, I need to tell you something."

Giselle's heart dropped into her stomach. So, there WAS something amiss. Her next thought was unnerving but predictable. *Oh God, he's married!* Drawing her own nervous breath, she decided to wait for an explanation. "Go ahead. What do you want to tell me?" she sighed.

"I had a health issue—a serious one," began Pete. He went on to explain the long hospital stay, the physical deterioration, the false alarms for finding a new heart, and the danger of almost dying when matches were unavailable. In short, everything spilled out. For Pete, there was a feeling of catharsis now that he had told the truth and unloaded his story to Giselle.

But there was still a response to hear, and Pete sat nervously awaiting it.

"So, is everything working?" Perhaps Giselle was thinking about more than her date's heart, but she inquired about the normalcy of his life and functionality.

"Yes, but there is a scar," explained Pete, probably stating the obvious.

"Can I see it?" This time, she exclusively meant the scar.

What happened next was unexpected but left an indelible mark on their future.

"He unbuttoned what I considered to be the ugliest shirt ever to reveal the scar from his heart surgery," said Giselle, who appeared to be more concerned about the shirt than the incision reminder underneath it.

"She leaned over and kissed the top of my scar," said Pete. "That was it!"

There were still formalities to take care of. The following weekend, Pete took Giselle to meet his family, and everyone showed—Mom, Dad, all four sisters with their spouses and children. "Mom invited the whole gang," said Pete.

Giselle was shell-shocked. Stability was lacking in her family unit. She grew up in a divorced family, her siblings rarely communicated, and she moved 10 times in one 15-year period.

The language barrier did not help. "I felt self-conscious of my shyness and felt anxious that they would make fun of my English." Still, the initial meeting with the Radigan clan went well, and the whirlwind romance continued.

"Every weekend, I'd go to her house, or she would come to mine," said Pete. "I worked a lot, training during the week and racking up a lot of frequent flier miles."

As the winter holidays approached, Pete decided that another bold move was in order. "I went to the Diamond District (in Manhattan) and bought an engagement ring. I planned to propose in time for Christmas, so I called her right after Thanksgiving and said, "Let's go away before Christmas. Pick a place."

I felt unprepared for her answer and could not believe it when it came. "Niagara Falls."

"It had to be kismet," said Pete. "That was where my donor family was from," a fact that his new love was unaware of.

The proposal was equally memorable, if only for its moments of irony. "It rained the whole time we were there, but we decided to go to the Falls anyway. The fog cleared right as we arrived. It was like God cleared the sky so we could have a moment." And Pete hoped to capture the moment. "I saw a tourist, went up with my camera, and told him—I am about to get engaged. Could you take a picture?"

It felt challenging to get the Falls, bended knee, ring, and bride-to-be in the same frame, but the most important part of the day was accomplished. Giselle said yes.

The first call went to Ellen Radigan, as promised. "I always told my mother she would be the first to know," said Pete. "Do you want to talk to your future daughter-in-law?" Somewhere among Ellen's tears of joy, the question was never answered, but Giselle took the phone and the two conversed together as future mother-in-law and daughter-in-law.

The second call went to Janet, and she and Pete set up a lunch date. "We talked about the wedding and some things with TSI," said Pete.

Janet's front-row view of the engagement and wedding planning process was laid out in her own careful words. As it turned out, Ellen Radigan was not the first to learn of her son's engagement.

From Janet's Journal

"It was a warm autumn day in October. The telephone rang. "Oh, hi, Pete. How are you?" I asked.

He responded, "Hey, Jan. Giselle and I want to visit Niagara Falls. We plan to visit in December."

"Are you crazy?" I retorted. December is the worst time to see Niagara Falls since the weather is usually gloomy, snowy, or cold, you pick! Why not wait until it is nicer weather?"

Pete replied, "I want you to meet my new girlfriend, Giselle, who has never been to Niagara Falls." With sheer confidence, peace, and excitement in his voice, he said, "She is the one for me!!!"

"Pete, I'm excited for you!" I said.

Pete then went on to explain how he met Giselle. He was in a restaurant in New Jersey and saw an attractive Hispanic girl who was sitting at a table with friends. He went over to her table, looked at her, and said, "I am attracted to you. Here is my phone number if you want to call me." He went on to say, "I know my approach was a bit forward, but what did I have to lose?"

Acting like an overprotective parent and being aware of some past hurtful relationships, I asked, "So what makes her different from the other women you dated?" I did not want him to be hurt again. He had already gone through a lot already. New challenges arise in the dating scene being a heart recipient.

He posed the question to me, "How and when do you tell your date you are a heart recipient?"

We bantered back and forth for a while, as I questioned him. Teasing him I said, "You know some children need one mother, some need two. I am glad you realize I have a stake in this since I am mother number TWO!" We laughed, as we usually did.

Returning to a serious note, I expressed my happiness for him and looked forward to meeting Giselle. As I hung up the phone, I knew there was something else on his mind he had not shared with me.

A few days before the trip to Niagara Falls, Pete contacted me and invited me to go out to lunch with them after they visited Niagara Falls. At about 1:30 p.m. on that cold, wintry Saturday, I went to the motel where they were staying to pick them up and take them to the restaurant. While waiting for them to come down from their room, I shared with the male receptionist the reason for my visit and my relationship with Pete. He was awe-stricken as he stopped his work to hear our story. He could not believe it.

As Pete and Giselle rounded the corner, I ran up to Pete, hugged him, and was introduced to Giselle. After we arrived at the restaurant, we talked non-stop, directing the waitress to return several times to obtain our order. When I returned from the bathroom, Giselle and Pete sat across from each other holding hands. I looked down and saw the diamond on Giselle's finger and exclaimed, "You got engaged!!!"

I tried to contain my excitement for them, and then I realized the reason for their visit to Niagara Falls. I looked over at Pete, who had a smug expression on his face as if he had won. He had!!! I hugged them and said to Pete, "Why did you not tell me?" From that point on, we all became tearful with joy, excited for the future, with lots of conversation.

As we talked, he explained he wanted to get engaged in the same area where his heart was donated, and Giselle had chosen this spot, which was the perfect place to ask for Giselle's hand in marriage.

Pete explained the story like this. He and Giselle had gone to Niagara Falls, where he wanted to propose to her near the brink of Niagara Falls. It rained that day, so the pavement was wet. Pete planned on taking pictures. He introduced himself to the only other person there and asked him if he could take a picture of the two of them, telling this tourist of his intent to propose to Giselle on bended knee. In the meantime, Giselle grew tired of waiting for Pete and hollered, "Come on over, Pete, so we can get pictures of the Falls!"

As Pete returned to Giselle, he bent one knee on the wet pavement and asked the life-changing question, "Will you marry me?"

Giselle shrieked with joy, and with tears streaming down her cheeks, she replied, "YES!!!."

The tourist who snapped the picture and captured the moment smiled! As he returned the camera, he told the newly engaged pair, "You made my day!" After sharing his story, we all shared tears of joy due to the happiness of the occasion! I felt so happy that Pete found Giselle to share his life with.

Now there was a wedding to plan."

14

Wedding Bells and Another Miracle

Even by Irish standards, the celebration leading up to the Radigan nuptials was fun-filled and boisterous. After meeting the future bride and groom, Father Pat, who had once administered last rites to Pete, agreed to officiate the wedding.

The search for a reception was easier than expected given the short time frame. Giselle and Pete eyeballed the Battleground Country Club in Manalapan, New Jersey. The new couple, following sage advice, made sure to have the church booked first before searching for a reception site; however, there was a booking at Battleground on the wedding date. But fate would win the day, literally. The original booker changed plans, and the preferred date opened again.

Giselle's mother and sisters arrived from Brazil for the prenuptial party. The festivities were a bit crazy between the party bus, shots of Jack Daniels, the large family, noise, commotion, and sharing the room with a group of Pete's close friends and fellow heart transplant recipients.

The April before the May wedding, Janet received a wedding invitation. "I felt excited to fly to New Jersey the day before the wedding. As I arrived at the church, my eyes glanced at the three groomsmen who I previously met, standing outside. Pete and Giselle invited a few donor families, as well. It felt surreal. I just stood and stared!! How could this be and yet it was. All the groomsmen previously received heart transplants!!! The groomsmen and Pete bonded through their struggles together, helping each other along the way as they waited for a miracle and a second chance at life. As I stood there, I felt fully aware they would not be here if others had not said "yes" to donation following a tragic death. Of course, the wedding was beautiful. As I later entered the Country Club, Pete introduced me to several people as we socialized before dinner."

Pete and Giselle planned to provide a small gift to Janet as she sat at her assigned table. They chose to surround her with friends and medical staff that played a significant part in supporting Pete throughout the grueling process of waiting for a heart transplant and the subsequent recovery: Lynn Kossow, his primary care doctor, Joe and Carole Guidice (the lung transplant recipient and his wife), and his good friends, Hans and Michele Schumacher. Joe received Tom's lung at the same time Peter received his heart.

> "I felt relieved to be sitting at the same table as Carole and Joe since I knew few people. As the evening progressed and the food arrived, everyone introduced themselves around the table. Dr. Kossow, his primary care physician who initially diagnosed him, sat next to me. Across the table sat Pete's friends who provided undue support to him throughout his wait. It felt amazing to see Pete's relatives, neighbors, friends, business partners, celebrating with them having supported him throughout his ordeal. I represented the other side of the equation, unbeknown to most everyone there."

"A small petite woman entered the reception area to sit at our table. The three groomsmen who were heart recipients rushed toward her, welcoming her. Dr. Mancini had arrived. She managed the medical care of all these heart recipients. Although petite in size, she carried a lot of authority and importance in the success or failure of their heart transplants. They could call her day or night and she responded immediately. She adjusted their medication or whatever other medical needs she could meet. She represented their harbor in the storm. Now, I planned to meet her. I cannot explain it. In one sense, it felt overwhelming, yet in another sense, it felt beautiful. As I introduced myself to her as the donor family, she thanked me as I reciprocated, thanking her for maintaining Pete's life that came from my son."

At 10:30, the DJ announced, "Pete has one last request" as he asked the curious onlookers, "Would Janet Mauk, the woman who made this possible, please approach the dance floor?" Surprised, Janet made her way to the center of the room where the lyrics of "Hero" by Mariah Carey began to resonate over the tired, but inquisitive crowd. Pete and the guests waited for his dance partner to reach the center of the dance floor. As the lyrics extolled the themes of heroism, strength and overcoming fear, for the next four minutes, it would become Janet Mauk's song as they danced together.

"As I arrived at the dance floor, the guests immediately stood up, gathered around the perimeter of the dance floor with tears streaming down their faces as the words of the song echoed in their ears. Initially, there became a resounding standing ovation!! Then a resounding quietness followed as people stood in silence, staring at us. Just as I stared at those groomsmen and friends who supported him throughout his journey, now they stared at me wondering if this was real, yet knowing it was. Those around the dance floor supported Pete throughout his circuitous physical path to health, not knowing if he would live or die. Now he celebrated his marriage to Giselle. Life had been passed on by saying 'yes' to donation and God's Will, giving Pete a second chance at life so he could celebrate life as he did before. Three small letters spell life. Saying 'Y-E-S' can provide life for others, a chance TOM would never have. My heart was full as I celebrated this momentous occasion with them."

And there, in the middle of the dance floor in front of at least 100 spectators, the room fell silent, as she heard and felt the heartbeat of her son, Tom.

> "As I returned to my table, several people huddled around to emotionally express their deep appreciation to me through tears as they hugged me. They admired my courage during the darkest day of my life. Others stated that, as a result, their lives drastically changed, too. They decided if, given the opportunity, they would donate their organs so they could save lives, as well."

The wedding was a combination of tradition tinged with old-fashioned Irish good luck. It was notable because of the presence of Pete's fellow transplant recipients. Frank Bodino served as the best man, and the other two groomsmen, Ed Masol and Don Arthur had also received the miraculous gift of life.

Following another Irish tradition, the oldest living relative gave a toast, and Pete's grandmother and family matriarch, Helen McGahan, 94 years young, raised a vase filled with beer to take the ceremonial first drink from what was called, "The Vase of Life." It was a tradition that started at his cousin's wedding. Pete's Uncle Ed (his mom's brother) got tired of getting up to get more beer, so he emptied the vase from the flower arrangement, cleaned it, and filled it with beer. Ceremoniously, the vase was sent around for everyone to take a sip of "The Vase of Life." The next wedding was Pete's sister, Jean, and she had a vase engraved "the Vase of Life" and Pete's grandmother, Helen McGahan, always took the first sip as the matriarch.

> "As I left the reception to return to the motel, a flicker of self-pity flashed in my mind for a few short minutes, but then the peace of giving life took over and I knew Tom's legacy continued."

Another Miracle - And then there were three...

Pete and Giselle Radigan were anxious to start building their family unit. For Pete, having a large family was an extension of his childhood, having grown up with four younger sisters at 16 Wickham Lane, East Windsor, New Jersey. They enjoyed large holiday gatherings, pool parties, and other family celebrations. He remembered one memorable party that occurred in May 1987 when Pete graduated from Wagner College, and Ellen used the occasion to double up and celebrate Tracey's Hightstown High Rams basketball team, which had won the New Jersey Group IV state championship with a 59-39 win over Bloomfield in the tournament final. From two in the afternoon to two in the morning, dozens of the Radigan family and friends laughed, swam, drank, cheered, and talked.

Giselle had bought into the idea of family expansion. While four of her family members had attended her wedding, there were fewer occasions for her family to talk and have fun. Her parents were divorced, and as she recalled, her parents and siblings were "not in each other's business."

Pete and Giselle decided it was time for yet one more miracle. Four years had passed since they were married, and the young couple's dream of starting a family remained unfulfilled and they decided it was time. Over the next few weeks, they tried to get pregnant. Two weeks later, Giselle showed Pete a positive pregnancy test. He was at once super excited and nervous at the same time. However, in the end, excitement won out.

Pete, with his usual dark sense of humor, proclaimed, "Two weeks and you are pregnant…What fun is that?"

"On October 2, 2007, our son was born. He comes from four generations of the same name. My full name is Edmund Peter Radigan. However, his grandfather was Edmund Peter Radigan, but they called him Bud. My father's name was the same, but they called him Mickey. Now my full name. The name had already been chosen, and Pete passed along his own middle name and the first name of his favorite cousin.

A birth certificate was drawn up, and Pete decided to pass along the news to his "second" mother, Janet Mauk.

"Giselle had a baby!" he exclaimed over the phone, having reached Janet in Niagara Falls.

"That's wonderful, Pete," said his excited friend. "What did you name it?"

Completely oblivious to the irony and the meaning, Pete replied, "Peter Thomas Radigan!" He was stunned when Janet's joy turned to silence.

"Is something wrong?"

The response ricocheted back in a subdued, almost hushed tone. "Did you do that on purpose?"

The past nine months had been a joyful and chaotic time for Pete and Giselle. In fact, their entire life together had been a whirlwind of activity, with his sales education job eventually forcing nine relocations in 15 years. He paused in reflection. "Peter…. Thom.."

The next verbal pause was his own. He could not have named his own son Thomas and not realize it was the same name as the New York teenager whose heart saved his life.

Pete gasped as the wheels of his mind moved quickly, hoping, and praying for a meaningful reply. What came out instead was the truth. "I wish I could tell you I did this on purpose." Another pause followed. "I thought of my cousin. All I can tell you is God works in mysterious ways."

Janet never expected that they would name their son Thomas, so she was surprised when she heard the news from Pete. She felt joyful for all of them.

For Pete Radigan, his life extension was like a highway, his highway of extended life. As with any highway, there are always bumps or potholes in the road. Pete has done a masterful job of caring for the precious gift Tom gave him. He avoids people who are sick but, in general, stays involved and lives life to the fullest. In reality, he has had hospital stays over the years, but sometimes all it takes is a positive attitude. But after 24 years, and with the lifesaving gift of Tom Mauk's heart, one undeniable fact is true, receiving the Gift of Life now afforded him a marriage, a son, and 24 years of life that may not have ended that way if Tom's parents did not say yes to donation. Three simple letters spell YES and they spell LIFE.

As Tom's legacy continues, we hope that donation is not as obscure as it once was, and it is more the norm than the exception. Our hope is others will say yes to donation if a tragedy should occur. Educating the public will, hopefully, result in more lives being saved and enhanced.

Epilogue

Cardiac transplantation has often been described as a miracle of modern medicine. It is a transformative procedure that literally restores life to a patient on the brink of death. It may sound melodramatic, but there are few fields in medicine where death and life are so closely juxtaposed. As a transplant cardiologist, I have had the privilege of participating in hundreds of these "little miracles" during my career and one of these little miracles involved Edmund 'Pete' Radigan.

I first met Pete over 20 years ago when he presented to Columbia Presbyterian Center as a young man with dilated cardiomyopathy and advanced heart failure. His heart failure quickly progressed, and he was hospitalized and supported with intravenous medication to await cardiac transplantation. The UNOS (United Network of Organ Services) donor allocation system at that time required all patients on parenteral inotropes to remain hospitalized awaiting transplant with continuous telemonitoring.

As donor scarcity has been a consistent obstacle to heart transplantation and as the era of durable mechanical support was still in its early stage, it meant patients waited weeks to months for a heart in the hospital. In many ways, these patients were like prisoners of war in a battle for survival. As a physician, you learned quite a lot about the patients, their families, and social support. During Pete's long wait for a transplant, it was apparent that he was determined to survive and to make the best possible use of his time. To this day I remember him vividly hard at work on his computer, learning, researching, and preparing for the next chapter of his life. He was a leader of the group of patients on the medical floor awaiting transplants and a constant support to them and their families. Most patients struggle with frustration over the long wait, and Pete did as well, but he was stoic; and with the strong support of his lovely family, he weathered this trying time.

His heart transplant went smoothly, and he rapidly recovered and was discharged. His return to "normalcy" was quick given his young age and lack of associated medical problems. With two fellow heart transplant recipients, Pete worked to organize a program to educate the public about heart transplantation and the need for organ donation. He traveled the country speaking on behalf of this cause.

His career also took him on a journey through many cities and transplant centers. He married, and one of my most pleasant memories was having the joy of dancing at his wedding. He became a dad. Of course, his post-transplant course was not without some medical problems.

Pete did develop atrial tachyarrhythmias and had syncopal episodes that resulted in hospitalizations and medical procedures, but those issues were treatable, and life was pretty much normal. During this time, he was also found to have Emery Dreifuss muscular dystrophy, which was probably the cause of his original cardiomyopathy. Dreifuss is a condition that primarily affects muscles used for movement (skeletal muscles) and the heart (cardiac muscle).

Many diseases will affect different body organs at different rates. For Pete, cardiomyopathy was the early manifestation of this inherited genetic defect. It is only due to the long-term success of his heart transplant, that other symptoms of muscular dystrophy have started to manifest in other organs like his respiratory and skeletal muscles.

Pete has been a warrior, a patient who has achieved a normal life, a survivor through all life's challenges. He continues to make the best of each day with each beat of his heart. On 8/5/97, he received his "Gift of Life" and with that gift, he has gone forward and given back so much to so many. Bravo, Pete!!!

- Dr. Donna Mancini - Cardiologist, Mount Sinai Hospital, New York City

About Transplant Speakers International (1999-2016)

Transplant Speakers International, Inc. (TSI) was created by a group of donor families and transplant recipients. Its sole mission was to create an organization that raised public awareness of organ donors and transplants so well that, in time, the need for the group would become obsolete.

TSI's Board was composed of educators who had been impacted by transplantation. Many are donor families who, through a family tragedy, gave the ultimate gift...the gift of life. Others have gone through the trauma of having a major organ or tissue fail and have become transplant recipients themselves.

Their personal stories, along with the experiences of all of the board members, led to the formation of TSI. TSI works hand-in-hand with organ procurement organizations, private organizations, and anyone whose mission includes public education on organ and tissue donation.

TSI is unique in the field of organ and tissue donation education, blending traditional instructor-led training programs with an exciting e-based learning package.

During its existence, TSI trained approximately 8,000 transplant recipients to share their stories with others over an 18-year period between 1999 and 2016. Their work led to speakers traveling as far as Hawaii, Newfoundland, England, and most of the continental United States.

Some of its teachings include:

Organ Donation: Names, Faces & Facts

TSI created this unique training offering to match its philosophy that until you put names, faces, and personalities with organ and tissue donation, it remains just a statistic in the minds of the public. This program was designed for schools with a strong administrative back end.

Volunteer Training

This program was designed to aid donor families, transplant recipients, or anyone whose mission included public education to speak effectively on organ and tissue donation. This program focuses on putting a narrative together, story writing, and letter writing to donor families and transplant recipients.

A Sorrowful Joy - A Donor Family Seminar

• Facilitated by high-profile donor family members.

• Donor family members speak on the healing effects of speaking about their experiences in a way that only a donor family can.

• Education on how to leave a legacy for their loved ones through speaking.

• Seminars are usually conducted just prior to TSI's Phase I and Phase II Educational Program.

OPO Staff Development I

• Designed for, but not limited to OPO Hospital Development, Clinical Staff Members, and Community Education Staff.

• Top-Down Approaching.

• Designing meeting goals utilizing outlining and prioritizing techniques.

• Proactive management techniques vs. reactive management techniques.

In its early stages and before Pete and Janet met, the original group of TSI's eight speakers presented Dr. Mehmet Oz, who Frank Bodino remembered "was the doctor for all eight of us," with a token of their appreciation. Oz, who was a proponent and donor to TSI, was given a plaque showing a hand holding a heart and surrounded by stones.

Appendix: How the donation process works - from Connectlife.org (formerly UNYTS)

A potential donor has most likely been admitted to a hospital because of illness or accident which has resulted in head trauma, brain aneurysm, or stroke. Healthcare professionals work hard to save the patient's life while maintaining the patient on mechanical devices.

Brain Death Testing

When healthcare professionals have exhausted all possible life-saving efforts and the patient is not responding, a physician will perform a series of tests to determine if brain death has occurred. This is usually done by a neurosurgeon in compliance with accepted medical practice and state law. Patients who are brain dead have no brain activity and cannot breathe on their own. Brain death is irreversible and is not a coma. Brain death is death.

Alerting ConnectLife

In compliance with federal regulations, a hospital notifies its local organ procurement organization, ConnectLife, of every death or impending death. A hospital gives ConnectLife information about the deceased to confirm his or her potential to be a donor. If the patient is a potential candidate for donation, a representative from ConnectLife immediately travels to the hospital.

Obtaining Authorization

The ConnectLife representative will search New York's donor registry to see if the deceased had enrolled as a donor. If so, the person's consent will serve as legal authorization. If the deceased has not registered and there was no other legal authorization for donation, ConnectLife will seek authorization from the individual of highest decision-making priority. When authorization is obtained, a medical evaluation will continue, including obtaining the deceased's complete medical and social history from the family.

Matching Donors with Recipients

If the deceased's evaluation does not rule out donation, ConnectLife will contact the Organ Procurement and Transplantation Network (OPTN) to begin the search for matching recipients. A computer program matches donor organs with recipients based on blood type, tissue type, height and weight, length of time the patient has been waiting, the severity of the patient's illness, and the distance between the donor's and the recipient's hospitals. The list does not reference race, gender, income, or social status.

Maintaining the Donor

While the matching process is happening, the donor is maintained on artificial life support and the condition of each organ is carefully monitored by the hospital medical staff and the Clinical Donation Coordinator from ConnectLife.

Recovering and Transporting Organs

The ConnectLife representative arranges the arrival and departure times of the transplant surgical teams. After the surgical team arrives, the donor is taken to the operating room where organs and tissues are recovered in a sterile environment, just like in any surgery. All incisions are surgically closed and should not interfere with an open-casket funeral.

Transplanting Organs

The transplant operation takes place after the transport team arrives at the recipient hospital with the new organ. Typically, the transplant patient is already at the hospital and may be in the operating room awaiting the arrival of the lifesaving organ. Surgical teams work around the clock as needed to transplant the new organs into the waiting recipients.

Family Care

The families of all donors and potential donors are provided support through the ConnectLife Family Services departments. (https://www.connectlife.org/services/donor-family-services).

To Remember Me

The day will come when my body will lie upon a white sheet neatly tucked under four corners of a mattress located in a hospital busily occupied with the living and the dying. At a certain moment, a doctor will determine that my brain has ceased to function and that, for all intents and purposes, my life has stopped.

When that happens, do not attempt to instill artificial life into my body by the use of a machine. And don't call this my death bed. Let it be called the Bed of Life, and let my body be taken from it to help others lead fuller lives. Give my sight to the man who has never seen a sunrise, a baby's face, or love in the eyes of a woman. Give my heart to a person whose own heart has pain. Give my blood to the teenager, who was pulled from the wreckage of his car, so that he might live to see his grandchildren play. Give my kidneys to one who depends on a machine to exist from week to week. Take my bones, every muscle, every fiber and nerve in my body and find a way to make a crippled child walk. Explore every corner of my brain. Take my cells, if necessary and let them grow so that someday, a speechless boy will shout at the crack of a bat and a deaf girl will hear the sound of rain against her window. Burn what is left of me and scatter the ashes to the winds to help the flowers grow. If you must bury something, let it be my faults, my weaknesses, and all prejudice against my fellow man.

Give my sins to the devil, give my soul to God. If, by chance, you wish to remember me, do it with a kind deed or word to someone who needs you. If you do all I have asked, I will live forever.

Robert N.Test

The Cincinnati Post

The National Donor Registry

Deceased organ donation is the process of giving an organ or a part of an organ, at the time of the donor's death, for the purpose of transplantation to another person. At the end of your life, you can give life to others.

In order for a person to become an organ donor, blood and oxygen must flow through the organs until the time of recovery to ensure viability. This requires that a person die under circumstances that have resulted in a fatal brain injury, usually from massive trauma resulting in bleeding, swelling or lack of oxygen to the brain.

Only after all efforts to save the patient's life have been exhausted, tests have been performed to confirm the absence of brain or brainstem activity, and brain death has been declared, is donation a possibility.

The state and national Donate Life Registries are searched securely online to determine if the patient has personally authorized donation. If the potential donor is not found in the Registry, his or her next of kin or legally authorized representative (usually a spouse, relative or close friend) is offered the opportunity to authorize the donation. Once the donation decision is established, the family is asked to provide a medical and social history. Donation and transplantation professionals determine which organs can be transplanted and to which patients on the national transplant waiting list the organs are to be allocated.

Why register your decision to be a donor?

By registering your decision to be an organ, eye and tissue donor in the National Donate Life Registry, you are helping to save lives and give hope to the more than 100,000 people in the United States currently waiting for lifesaving organ transplants. Thousands more people are in need of tissue or corneal transplants to restore health. One donor can save and heal more than 75 lives. **Register TODAY: RegisterMe.org**

The National Donate Life Registry

Donate Life America manages the National Donate Life Registry.

Registering your decision to be an organ donor in the National Donate Life Registry ensures your donor registration travels with you, no matter where you live or move across the country.

When you register in the National Donate Life Registry, you are registering to be an organ, eye and tissue donor for the purpose of saving and healing lives through transplantation.

There are currently more than 7.3 million donor registrations in the National Donate Life Registry.

How it works

You can register in the National Donate Life Registry at RegisterMe.org, in your iPhone Health App or using our on-site registration form.

Any adult age 18 or older can register to be an organ, eye and tissue donor – regardless of age or medical history. 15-17 year olds can register their intent to be organ, eye and tissue donors in the National Donate Life Registry. However, until they are 18 years old, a parent or legal guardian makes the final donation decision. If registering in the National Donate Life Registry through iPhone, you must be 18 years or older.

Your *privacy* is important. We work to make sure personal data is safe, secure and protected. Donate Life America may disclose registration information to other entities, such as recovery agencies, solely for the purpose of recognizing and acting on your donation decision at the time of your death.

DonateLife.net/types-of-donation/deceased-donation/

DonateLife.net/national-donate-life-registry/

The National Living Donor Registry

Living organ donation offers another choice for some transplant candidates, reducing their time on the waiting list and leading to better long term outcomes for the recipient.

The Need

A living donor is an option for patients who otherwise may face a lengthy wait for an organ from a deceased donor. To spare an individual a long and uncertain wait, relatives, loved ones, friends, and even individuals who wish to remain anonymous may serve as living donors.

Kidney and liver transplant candidates who are able to receive a living donor transplant can receive the best quality organ much sooner, often in less than a year.

• More than 100,000 people are on the national transplant waiting list.

• More than 85% of patients waiting are in need of a kidney.

• 11% of patients waiting are in need of a liver.

• In 2020, 5,700 more lives were saved through the generosity of living donors.

Facts about Living Donation

Want to learn more about living donation? Here are some key facts:

• Living donation is an opportunity to save a life while you are still alive.

• Living organ donation and transplantation was developed as a direct result of the critical shortage of deceased donors.

• Living donors don't have to be related to their recipients. On average, 1 in 4 living donors are not biologically related to the recipient.

• Patients who receive a living donor transplant are removed from the national transplant waiting list, making the gift of a deceased donor kidney or liver available for someone else in need.

If you are considering being a living donor, it's important to note that living donation is not included in your deceased donor registration. In 2022, you will be able to register your interest in being a living donor in the National Donate Life Living Donor Registry (visit DonateLife.net for updates). A living donor transplant program will conduct a full evaluation to determine your eligibility to be a living donor.

The National Donate Life Living Donor Registry

In an effort to streamline the living donation process and help save more lives, DLA is currently working with funding partner, Fresenius Medical Care Foundation, to develop the National Donate Life Living Donor Registry. Launching in 2022, the Living Donor Registry will allow individuals to register their interest in being a living kidney donor and receive a preliminary at-home testing kit to help with further evaluation by a living donor transplant program. Visit DonateLife.net for updates.

DonateLife.net/types-of-donation/living-donation/

BIOMATRIX]

BioMatrix is a transplant focused specialty pharmacy dedicated to the unique needs of the transplant community. Tragedy to Triumph is an inspiring story demonstrating the incredible power of transplant. We supported this book to help Janet and Pete share their exceptional story and raise awareness about the importance of organ donation. BioMatrix supports solid organ, tissue, and eye transplant patients across the transplant continuum of care. Our multidisciplinary team works as an extension of the transplant center, excelling in support for highly sensitized patients, patients experiencing chronic or acute transplant complications, and standard of care immunosuppressive medications. Our clinicians are advancing the science of transplant through clinical trials and research addressing critical issues across the transplant journey. We understand the life-changing importance of organ donation and work to achieve favorable outcomes across the transplant continuum of care.

To learn more visit: https://www.biomatrixsprx.com/transplant

SUPPORTERS

These supporters and many more like them save lives every day. Please join us in thanking our sponsors below.

Children's Organ
Transplant Association

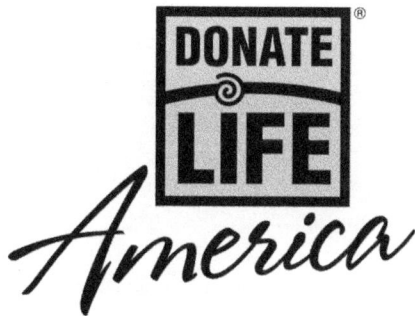

DONATE
LIFE
America

BIOMATRIX

TRANSPLANT NEWS

Acknowledgements

The authors wish to thank the sponsors who recognized the uniqueness of this book and its ability to show that in tragedy there can be hope. All of the sponsors in their individual ways support organ, eye, and tissue donation. Thank you for all you do!

www.ingramcontent.com/pod-product-compliance
Lightning Source LLC
Chambersburg PA
CBHW030503210326
41597CB00013B/779